One Brief Shining Moment

12/1/01

To Lee,
I hope you enjoy
this. It wasn't an
easy thing to do, but
worth it.

One Brief Shining Moment

Ariene C. Swirsky

Writers Club Press
San Jose New York Lincoln Shanghai

One Brief Shining Moment

Writers Club Press
an imprint of iUniverse.com, Inc.

For information address:
iUniverse.com, Inc.
5220 S 16th, Ste. 200
Lincoln, NE 68512
www.iuniverse.com

ISBN: 0-595-17031-5

Printed in the United States of America

Youth and stupidity are synonymous. There is, in youth, an implicit trust in prevailing justice. Sometimes it is actually possible to accept the belief in the existence of a benevolent god. As you grow, the unthinkable concept of reality is defined.

When you are young, you are certain that everything you create is cloaked in a protective mantle and that nothing bad can penetrate its armor. In the master plan, there are no obstacles that cannot be overcome. Experience forces you to acknowledge of the difference.

As you grow, there is a realization that it is probably better not to have known about the future. Maybe the master plan is to simply keep you stupid.

Twenty-nine years ago is a long time in the past for me to try to remember, particularly, when all I want is to remember it in a different way.

Chapter One

There was a Sunday morning, twenty-nine years ago, I remember so very clearly. It was warm still, as the September sun had just begun to break through the dawn haze. The relative humidity was high enough to kink my hair and make me look like a stand-in for Little Orphan Annie. I felt fat, my usual weight of 100 pounds had ballooned to a massive one fifteen by the end of this pregnancy and made me feel like something that had washed up on the beach at low tide. At only five feet one inch, the disproportionate weight dispersal tended to throw off my balance. That morning, I was more than a little astonished when I felt the early throes of labor: my first child kept me dangling almost two extra weeks beyond my due date. This baby was going to do everything right, he or she was going to be on time and cooperate. I sat up in bed, determined to wait until I was sure this was, in fact, in labor; false alarms are embarrassing. This was one lesson I had learned two years previous in Tarrytown, New York, when I thought I might have been in labor. Having terrific stomach pains, upon arrival at the hospital I got an enema and a full prep, because the on-call doctor in the emergency room was a dermatologist and couldn't tell the difference between labor pains and gas pains. He had put his hand on my stomach and pronounced in a voice too loud, "this woman is in labor."

When four weeks later I was in labor and the lovely prep job of shaving me from chest to thighs had finally begun to grow back in, the labor nurse came in to prep me again, looked at my stubble and asked "Do you do this sort of thing regularly?"

After two full hours had passed and things seemed to be moving along nicely, I woke Bruce out of a seemingly pleasant snoring episode at the crack of eight a.m. We called the doctor, called my in-laws to baby-sit for Alyssa, had a bite of breakfast, took my little suitcase and left for Worcester Hahnemann Hospital. So far so good.

My in-laws, Carl and Sylvia met us at Hahnemann and took Alyssa out for breakfast, while we checked in. Quintessential Jewish grandparents, Carl and Sylvia doted on Alyssa. They loved spending time with her and plying her with potato latkes, bagels, cream cheese and lox.

Alyssa had started speaking in clear sentences at the age of one, and by the lofty age of two, there was no preventing her from voicing her opinions. We used to joke that she was born to be a lawyer, as only a judge could silence her arguments. She didn't know what was happening that morning, but she was delighted Papa was taking her to spend a day with him and Gramma. She knew this meant treats, toys and jumping all over him without the constraint of her parents telling her to stop because Papa was getting tired.

No sooner had I been admitted and situated in the labor suite, when my labor stopped. Still I tried to remain unconcerned. No problem. The obstetrician came in to check me out. He again assured us everything was as it should be. Twenty-nine years ago, male doctors assumed all of their female patients were dense and all trusting. I guess we were. He scampered out of the labor suite, with Bruce in tow, and congratulated him on the impending birth of his second daughter, neglecting to tell me that my latest bundle of joy was in a frank breech position. That kind of information he deemed "need to know"; why panic a mother before you absolutely had to was the prevailing medical prudence and procedure of the day. He assured Bruce again, everything was under control, and I probably still could deliver her naturally with neither medication nor complications. He wanted to simply restart my labor with pitocin and get things moving along.

The two of them trooped into the labor room dressed in scrubs, and my obstetrician told me he was going to have the nurses run some pit into my I.V. get my labor moving. Bruce looked ridiculous in the scrubs that only reached half way down his pole-vault long legs and to the forearms of his 36 inch-long arms. The silly-looking surgical cap came nowhere near covering all of his wavy black hair, and having not shaved that morning; the mask kept getting stuck on his black stubby chin. Still no word to me about my rear-facing daughter. I would have to figure that one out when the time came.

When the contractions started up again, they were unrelenting and severe. Not five minutes after they inserted the I.V., and started the pitocin drip I was on the way to delivery. Two years before I had gone through the same kind of thing, or so I thought. I knew there was nothing to worry about. I knew what to expect as far as what came out first, how long it took for the rest of the baby to appear, how long it would take until the mouth kicked in, all of the good stuff. The nurses would laugh and joke around and then proclaim what a beautiful child you had. They would comment on the amount of, or the lack of hair. The doctor would congratulate Bruce and me for doing such a wonderful job of coaching and pushing respectively. It would be a very happy place indeed.

After twenty minutes of accelerating contractions, the doctor told me to go ahead and push. Looking in the overhead mirror, the first things I saw were feet.

"Holy Shit! It's breech! Why didn't you tell me?"

The doctor explained that he thought that it would be too stressful for me if I knew. He wanted me relaxed so that I could deliver from the breech position naturally. Well, that made sense. I had been told that even though I was very short and thin, the internal width of my pelvis would have allowed me to deliver a small elephant and still have room to spare, why get all upset and nervous. Following the feet and legs out slid hips, chest, arms and finally the head. The baby was a girl. She had black hair, and looked like a normal, wrinkly baby except for one thing: nothing happened.

She did not move. She did not cry. Her color was a sickly looking, dusky gray-blue. Do not panic yet, I tried to tell myself, breech babies are frequently a little sluggish at birth, I had read. The attention instantly shifted focus from me to the baby, as they suctioned her nose and mouth, and finally we got a weak little cry.

"What's wrong?" I screamed. But nobody said anything. "What the hell is going on here?"

It became deathly soundless in the delivery suite. They wanted to get the house pediatrician in to check her out immediately, but she seemed somewhat stable at that moment. Probably just worn out from the trauma of the delivery, they assured me. The platitudes worked, mainly because I wanted them to. In light of what she had been through, the obstetrical nurse said, she looked all right. We all calmed down a little bit.

Chapter Two

The only resemblance we saw to Alyssa were the mop of black hair, and the jet black eyes, but she was not the healthy looking, red-faced, screeching infant her sister had been. I remembered that Alyssa looked like an angry Navaho Indian and sounded as if someone had given her a hotfoot as a newborn, while this baby hardly moved and made no sounds.

When one has just finished delivering a child, something strange happens. All of my friends have mentioned that after delivery they too felt cold and needed heated blankets to warm up, as I had, two years before. But this time I was shaking so uncontrollably that no matter how many blankets they piled on top of me, I could not stop trembling.

When I was finally stitched up and taken to my room, and Bruce had gone to call all of the family and friends, I talked myself into believing all was fine and normal. My obstetrician came in and put on his comforting face. He had delivered scores of breech babies: many of them were slow getting started. It was, he said, because that kind of delivery was so intense and traumatic for the baby. Still, he said, she was much better off because there were no drugs in my system, she was full term, and her weight of six pounds four ounces was fine. The house pediatrician thought it made sense to keep her in the nursery for a few hours so the house staff could keep a collective eye on her. My private pediatrician, whom I had yet to meet, would be in to evaluate the baby within the hour. As we were in the process of moving into a new home, I had only just contacted the new pediatrician a week or two before my due date.

Some time that afternoon, after Bruce had left to pick up Alyssa, they brought the new baby in to me to feed. I put the bottle in her mouth and waited for something to happen. I stroked her little cheek and still nothing happened. All this baby wanted to do was sleep. I rocked her for a little while, and then remembered the easiest way to wake a newborn was to undress it. I started to peel off the blanket. Still sleeping. I took off her little shirt. I took off the diaper. Still nothing. This child needed a serious nap, I thought. I redressed her and tried to feed her again. Nothing yet. A huge nurse, who looked as if she would have been more comfortable in marine fatigues and combat boots, strode into the room.

"What's the matter with you? Don't you know how to feed a baby?" The "you idiot," was implicit in her tone.

I handed over my baby and sat there and watched her as she met with the same lack of success that I had.

"I guess I don't know how to feed a baby." I replied.

She tried the same tricks I had. She uncovered the baby's feet and pinged the bottoms of her feet trying to wake her up.

"Sleepy baby, isn't she." The more nervous I became the more the lifelong tendency to become smart-mounted tended to show up. That day was no exception.

The "powers that be," decided that it would be in her best interest to keep her in the nursery and gavage feed her. They explained to me that whenever they wanted to feed her, they would insert a size 10 French catheter into her nose, thread it through her esophagus, then into her stomach and pour the formula slowly down the tube into her stomach. I had to admit this whole procedure sounded frightful and scared the hell out of me, but I gave my consent and permission to treat, as she had to receive some nutrition, and there was definitely something wrong with the way she sucked and swallowed.

Late that evening, Dr.John Tkach, knocked on the door and entered my room. He was the pediatrician I was waiting to meet. In his suit and tie, with glasses perched on the end of his nose, carrying charts and books under his arm, he looked more like an accountant than a pediatrician.

"I expected you sooner," I snapped.

Although his manner was somewhat terse, he told me he had spent two hours with my child earlier in the day, and that he had only just finished his evening rounds. As our relationship grew through the years, I came to understand this man's immense amount of devotion to his patients, not to mention his enormous compassion for the parents of his patients. His exceptional gifts were his gentle intelligence and perception, not his initial tact.

"Your daughter seems to have a problem."

No shit Sherlock, I thought, but had the good sense not to say.

"I am not sure what it is, but it seems almost impossible for her to swallow. Also, her reflexes are practically nonexistent. I have called in an E.N.T. and a pediatric neurologist to evaluate her. I have never seen anything like this before, but with a little bit of luck, we should be able to handle it. It is most likely some kind of developmental anomaly. If I had not read your chart, I would have sworn that this is baby was premature. Developmentally she is at the level of a seven or eight month fetus."

"I don't understand."

"Neither do I," he said simply. "There are certain little signs one always sees in preemies, some of which she has, like the lack of development of breast tissue, an unusual Babinsky reflex, that almost always indicate a lapse in fetal development. She seems to react as a preemie would but doesn't look like one. I have spoken to your obstetrician and he has assured me that you were at term."

"He also told me that you had a problem with bleeding in your third month. Tell me about it."

"My aunt, Lil, in New Jersey, had been hit by a car, and was killed. We drove down to New Jersey for the funeral, and I started to have some light bleeding and spotting. I stayed in New Jersey for a week, on Provera and the bleeding stopped. That was all that there was to it. Many women spot in their first trimester, they told me not to worry about it. Apart from that, the only other problem that I had was with very low blood sugar. But that also happened when I was pregnant with Alyssa, and she's fine."

"I want to do some more reading, and check on the baby in the morning. In the meantime, they are going to keep her in the nursery and feed her there." With that he left.

I cried all night.

Chapter Three

Things were not better in the morning. They were worse. She had still not awakened, and there was no discernable improvement in her ability to feed. I sat in my room staring out the windows, not wanting to eat and not talking. My roommate was mysteriously moved in to another room. Each time the nurses brought babies out of the nursery to their mothers, I wept. Mine only went to x-ray, or into a little examining room, behind the viewing nursery.

Laughter came from the other rooms on the floor. My door stayed shut. I could not stand that sound. Bruce came in three or four times a day to see our daughter and me. When he returned to the family business, a woman's clothing store, Carl and Sylvia came to see us, full of assurances and promises. My mother and brother called: I told them not to come up from New Jersey and North Carolina respectively until I asked them to. I did not want to see anyone. Friends came by, I did not want to see them and they did not know what to say. They did not stay long. What could anyone say? I started to smoke again. Days went by. Nothing improved.

We named her Heather Beth. Heather for Bruce's grandfather Harry, and Beth for my grandmother Bella. Now, if something happened, at least she would have a name. After five days, I went home, in time for Alyssa's second birthday. All of our friends came. Carl, Sylvia, my mother, Minna and my aunt Pauline drove up to help Alyssa celebrate. I did not feel much like celebrating; my second daughter was in hospital oblivion. No one had a clue as to what was wrong with her.

When she was eight days old, Heather opened her eyes for the first time, by herself. But, instead of bright, glistening eyes that babies normally have, hers were clouded over, grayish and hazy. I could not understand what the Hell was happening to us. They still had to tube feed her every two hours, she still had no reflexes, and now there was a problem with both of her eyes. None of this made any sense to me. She looked perfectly normal. She was losing the scrunched-up look that she had after the breech delivery; to look at her, one would never think that there were any problems. She was a good size, just over six pounds, had a mop of black silky curly hair, a fair porcelain complexion, and looked like a nice normal Gerber Baby Food illustration.

I had spoken to Dr. Tkach several times a day. On the ninth day, he told me that he wanted to send her to Mass General Hospital, in Boston. He had come up with a tentative, if rather bizarre diagnosis, and he asked the pediatric neurologists there to either confirm it, or diagnose her. The next morning we signed the necessary paperwork and into the ambulance went Heather, her nurses, the driver, and more equipment that I had ever seen attached to an isolette.

We followed the ambulance east on Route 9 then onto the Mass Turnpike into Boston, through the maze of early morning traffic, down Storrow Drive, off at Government Center, and into the ambulance bay of the Massachusetts General Hospital. Neither Bruce nor I spoke during the drive to Boston. We were not in the frame of mind to discuss or speculate about any of the horrific possibilities. We have always had a mysterious knack for knowing almost exactly what the other was thinking, and there was no question in either of our minds that we had to be ready for some fear-inspiring news. Silently, we each prepared for whatever it was they were going to tell us. What ever it was going to be, it was going to change our lives forever. They took Heather directly to the Newborn Intensive

Care Unit.

We went to admitting.

As the clerk filled out the admitting sheet, I tried to read the diagnosis on the upside down paper. It had more letters in it than I could handle from that angle. All I could make out was something that looked like FAMILY DYSAUT. When we had finished in admitting, we found our way up it the sixth floor. There, we were told to wait and a Dr. John Crawford would be with us as soon as possible.

Two hours later, a tall, thin, gray haired man, and a younger, stocky-looking man approached us. The gray haired man was Dr. Crawford, a pediatric neurologist. I did not catch the other man's name.

"You're Jewish, aren't you?"

That was a strange way to start this conversation, I thought. We answered together, "Yes."

"Did either of your mothers or grandmothers have a history of miscarriages?"

"I don't know." I had the feeling I was poorly prepared for a final exam.

"It appears that your child has a very, very rare genetic disease. It is called Familial Dysautonomia, an autonomic, neurological problem. It is one of the Jewish genetics diseases. I'll write it down for you."

He handed us a piece of paper, and we looked at it blankly. What does it mean? Will she outgrow it? Will it kill her? All of these questions ran through my mind at light speed, but I just sat there, mute.

"Although we have never had a case of this here," he continued......
WAIT ONE MINUTE!!RED LIGHT!! NO CASES AT MASS GENERAL!! WHAT THE HELL IS THIS!!! I started to feel that hot/cold, sick/dizzy out of control feeling you have just before throwing up or passing out.

"When Dr. Tkach called us with his tentative diagnosis, we had to do some reading, and I am confident we will be able to either confirm or deny his diagnosis rather quickly."

I knew I was going to be sick.

"Would you like to see your daughter before you leave? We will be working with her all night and there is no point in your staying. You'd just be in the way."

As we walked into the newborn ICU I felt myself begin to get light-headed. I had never been anywhere like this is my life. It was the most frightening place I had ever seen. We followed Dr. Crawford to the only normal looking child into the pediatric intensive care unit, Heather. I tried not to look at any of the other babies in the unit. Each of them was attached to some kind of massive machine, either breathing for them, or doing God knows what. Most of the birth defects these children had were patently obvious. One had a feeding tube surgically implanted in his thin belly, another looked like bones were missing from his arms and legs. A third baby was bluish and had a cardiac monitor pinging and sounding alarms alternately. Each baby, including mine, was attached to a cardiac monitor. I bent into Heather's isolette and kissed her cheek. Bruce, who was never very good at dealing with hospitals and stayed out of them whenever possible, was in a state of stunned shock and could not move. He stood, feet rooted to the floor in front of Heather's isolette and stared straight down at his new daughter.

We knew nothing about this disease. It wasn't until weeks later when I received the first of the myriad of literature about Familial Dysautonomia that I learned it was a Jewish genetic disease that affects the autonomic and central nervous systems. It is the autonomic system that controls all of the functions the human body does unconsciously. It controls blood pressure, heart rate, temperature, breathing, reflexes and the perception of pain, among many other things. There are hundreds of components of this system that all humans take for granted. These are the things Heather would never be able to rely upon to keep her body functioning normally. There were less than three hundred documented cases in the entire country. Many Dysautonomic children, I later learned, were either miscarried, died before they were diagnosed or misdiagnosed as an aberrant case of cerebral palsy, or some form of brain damage.

For four weeks, the routine was the same. I would get up in the morning, get Alyssa dressed so that Bruce could take her to his parent's house, and drive to Mass General. I swore many times that there was a special gear in my car that went straight to MGH. Most of the time I'd be on the Mass Pike with no recollection of how I got there. I found myself driving on autopilot. At night, we would have dinner together, play with Alyssa, pack up the apartment and collapse, exhausted by the strain of making it through another day. Most nights, we were asleep before we hit the bed. Our moving date was to be November 15.

The Newborn ICU was generally a quiet place. Those babies did not cry much. The radio played constantly, and by the time we left the unit, I knew all of the words to "THE NIGHT THEY DROVE OLD DIXIE DOWN" and "MAGGIE MAY." Whenever one of those songs would come on the radio everyone there would sing along through their work. Cardiac alarms were a staple of life in the unit. I got so familiar with the cardiac drill, that when one of the alarms went off, and the nurse assigned to that particular baby was busy, I would ping the soles of its tiny feet as I had seen them do so many times. That usually did the trick. There were some mornings when I got to the unit and one of the babies was gone. I learned, early, not to ask about what happened to them. For Heather, there were the never-ending neuro and ENT workups and more ophthalmologists than I knew existed in the western civilized culture. They evaluated her endlessly, administering all sorts of tests. There were two definitive diagnostic criteria for Dysautonomia: no taste buds on the tongue and an aberrant reaction to an intradermal histamine test. The intradermal histamine test is somewhat like an allergy test. The usual reaction is called a "wheal and flare", which means the injection causes a small swelling and there is generally redness around it. With dysautonomic children there is a wheal, but no flare. I was learning more medicine than I had ever wanted to know.

One of Heather's biggest problems was that her eyes were, for all practical purposes, totally dry. She produced no tears and the simple friction of her lids against her corneas was enough to abrade them. We devised a system of putting a special methylcellulose drops into her eyes every ten minutes or so, while she was awake. Had we not done this, she would have been blind in a matter of weeks from corneal abrasions, ulcerations and scarring.

The other big problem was feeding. The neurologists told me that my daughter had no reflexes whatever. That meant that when you put a bottle into her mouth, she could not reflexly suck or swallow as normal babies did. Also, she did not have a gag reflex, and frequently she would aspirate her food and it would wind up in a lung. Aspiration Pneumonia was to be a more frequent phrase in our vocabulary than common cold. We tried to teach her how to suck on a pacifier, and met with only modest success. I suggested that perhaps it would not be as much of a difficulty when she was able to eat solid food. They reminded me that another legacy of this wonderful disease, was that the children had no taste buds at all, and she would never be able to appreciate the flavor of anything. This promised to be the least of her problems.

I noticed that there seemed to be no direct response when they drew blood. She did not cry or seem to object very much when a tourniquet was placed around her arm. It was pointed out to me she also could not feel pain or perceive the difference between hot and cold. The doctors at Mass General spoon fed me little bits and pieces about this disease, and from what they told me, it seemed manageable, and certainly not necessarily life threatening or a real handicap.

I had called my older brother because I was having a problem finding information about this anomaly. As an Endocrinologist and pH. D. in physiology working for the US Public Health Service at the time he had access to a great many resources I did not. He had never heard of this rather unusual disease in either medical school or graduate school. He said he would check it out and send me whatever literature he could find.

By the time Heather was discharged, we had moved into our new house. It was a traditional split entry ranch with three bedrooms and a bath and a half. We had moved to the town of Paxton, a small bedroom community in Central Massachusetts, just west of Worcester. Somehow with the help of everyone we knew we were unpacked and organized. The house was freshly painted, new carpeting was down and every inch of the house was clean, scrubbed and in order. We hired a baby nurse to live in for two weeks to help with Heather while we finished the little things around the house and got Alyssa acclimated.

At the time of her discharge from Mass General, Dr. Crawford gave me two cautions. I have never forgotten them. 1. Do not let her fly in an unpressurized plane, and 2. Do not let her swim under water. They stand out in my mind, as both a grievous lack of information, and a sin of ignorance.

Chapter Four

Things were actually progressing. I found that if I fed Heather semi-solid foods, she could handle them without aspirating, most of the time. I had mastered the art of passing a gavage tube without too much trouble but every time I did, my hands shook and perspiration ran down my face and under my arms. There was always the possibility of putting the tube in wrong and having it wind up in a lung. Every time I passed a gavage tube I had to put the external end into a glass of water. If it bubbled, I was in a lung. Eventually I figured out that if I mixed rice cereal with formula to give it some body, then fed it through a bottle that had a nipple with a hole cut out to about one eighth inch in diameter, Heather could swallow it more easily.

The eyedrops were exhausting. We used a kitchen timer so we did not forget. Most of the time, she could manage with the drops every fifteen to twenty minutes. It did get to a point where life was approaching something that could almost be construed as normal. I was learning how to deal with this disease without allowing it to completely devastate my lifestyle. After all, hadn't Dr. Crawford said there were only two things I had to look out for? I certainly thought I could keep my daughter safe from unpressurized air travel, and when the time came, I would teach her how to swim safely, so she would not drown.

One afternoon, in November, the doorbell rang. It was the UPS delivery driver, no doubt another baby gift. The return address however, was US Public Health Service, and the package weighed about five pounds. I opened it and there was a note from my brother, saying something like, try not to read all of this at one time. I immediately sat down and read everything in the package, from beginning to end. The more I read, the more I firmly believed that this was some kind of sick joke. This morbid, death sentence surely could not be the same thing that Heather had. Clearly that was totally impossible. I read and tears ran silently down my cheeks. I read more. I cried more. I read and cried all afternoon.

This pile of good news told me that I could probably expect my daughter to spend much of her life in intensive care units, going from one kind of crisis to another, and the litany of possible crises was endless. Cyclic vomiting, every ten to twenty minutes for days to weeks. Blood pressure and temperature fluctuations that swung wildly from extreme highs to extreme lows in minutes. GI bleeds, seizures, physical limitations of growth and development, frequent accidents and trips to Emergency Rooms from fractures and lacerations caused from the lack of reflexes and pain recognition. Corneal ulceration and possible loss of sight from scarring, scoliosis frequent aspiration pneumonia; the list seemed endless. Then came the statistics: one in four children died before age five. After that, mortality increased. Almost none survived beyond adolescence. Out of every four pregnancies I might have, one child would have the disease, two would be carriers, and one would be normal. As Ashcanazic Jews, both Bruce and I had to carry the defective gene. There was no test to either diagnose prenatally, or screen for carriers. The incidence of learning disabilities increased if the child lived long enough to get into school, because of constant hospitalizations and absence. There were also speech and language difficulties. How could they not have told me any of this at Mass General?

I sat on the couch and read about my life to come and what I could expect from the devastating effects on my family, and I sobbed. I felt as I had gone through the looking glass.

By the time Bruce got home from the store I had been crying for hours. He listened as I summarized the information and he held me quietly. Somehow, we assured each other, we would survive this. We each had our strengths from which to draw. His were in his composure and ability to prioritize. Mine were still vague and shadowy, but showed some promise that I could learn from and assimilate the information that was going to become a huge measure of my daily existence.

As that first year unfolded we spent much time learning about ourselves and our ability to cope with problems. I learned I could live with more pressure than I had ever dreamed possible. I also learned how to switch gears on a dime, and go from a calm and relatively serene situation to total chaos while maintaining some semblance of control.

Although we had six or seven hospitalizations for pneumonia and bronchitis, nothing sticks out in my memory as one of the killers that first year. The highlights, or lowlights, were more along the lines of the creative problem solving variety. We noticed Heather had a peculiar penchant for sleeping with her eyelids only half shut. This became a disastrous condition, because we found we had to alternate staying up all night to put her eyedrops in. Believe me when I tell you that we were already at the limits of exhaustion before having to stay up all night. Our ophthalmologist was at a loss for a solution.

In the packet of literature my brother had sent were several reprints of articles published under the auspices of the DYSAUTONOMIA FOUNDATION in New York City. In desperation, I called them. It seemed this group was a repository of useful information that had been arrived at by other parents in desperate need of help dealing with a very extraordinary group of children. There was actually a treatment center at the NYU Med. Center in New York, and a doctor who had a patient base of more than one from which to draw. Dr. Felicia Axelrod was the personal savior of more than one hundred of these children and their exhausted parents. I called her.

Felicia set up an appointment for us at the New York University Medical Center in Manhattan to have Heather evaluated. In the meantime, she suggested that at night we put a heavy coating of Ilotycin, an antibiotic ophthalmic ointment into each of Heather's eyes, and then run a bead of the medication around each of her optic orbits, then cut rounds of Saran Wrap. These, we gently pressed over her eyes and formed individual moisture chambers. She looked strange as hell, but it worked.

Before we got to New York, Heather began to have violent episodes of retching in her sleep. The best way to describe them is by equating them to the dry heaves. Her tiny body would wrack and shake and her stomach would make regurgitive motions. It scared the hell out of me. I called John Tkach. He said he would talk to some other doctors and see if they had any beneficial suggestions. Needless to say, they did not. I called Felicia Axelrod. She told me that this was a variant of the cyclic vomiting and the best way to deal with it was by giving Heather either Valium or Thorazine before bedtime. We alternated these two medications until we could determine which was more effective and then added Thorazine to her nighttime repertoire. The Thorazine did not eliminate the nocturnal retching, but it did make the episodes less violent.

Exhaustion and stress were making Bruce and me tense and edgy. On top of this was the fear in the back of our minds about future children. We had always wanted three children, and had always wanted a boy, but circumstances made any thoughts of future pregnancies unrealizable. The genetics of Dysautonomia were clear: of every four pregnancies, one child would be born Dysautonomic, one would be totally free of the disease, and two of the four would carry the defective gene. There was no prenatal test or amniocentesis available, and there were no carrier screens. I had already begun to feel the dread of having to explain the odds and statistics to Alyssa when she was old enough to understand. It was hypothesized that approximately one of every 100 Ashcanazic Jews, whose ancestors had descended from the Jews who had migrated from the eastern part of Europe, carried this particular defective gene. Statistically it translated into an occurrence rate of 1/20,000 live births among Ashcanazic Jews.

I was becoming increasingly more apprehensive about the possibility of getting pregnant accidentally. I have always been a strong advocate of choice and was old enough to remember the back room horror stories of abortions performed with wire coat hangers that had led to the Rowe V. Wade decision. Forced to admit the knowledge that I could not take the chance of doing this to another innocent child and that my only option would then be abortion, Bruce and I decided that the only intelligent and responsible thing to do was to become incapable of further pregnancies. As much as I believed in choice and legal abortion, I did not think I personally could live with the reality of abortion. Of all of the choices a woman could conceivably make, this one had to be the most difficult and heart wrenching. My emotions had been contorted beyond their conceivable limits, and I did not think it could take any more dreadful decisions. Four months after Heather was born, with genetic counseling and much soul searching, I went back into the hospital, and had a tubal ligation.

Chapter Five

By the end of the first year, I had called John Tkach with so many bizarre symptoms he would have believed me if I told him that Heather was growing three heads and her hair was turning green.

Another little trick that started when Heather was about eighteen months old was sometimes when she got angry because she was frustrated, she would cry and forget to breathe. At that point she would have a tonic/clonic seizure, fall on the floor, hands postured backwards, feet splayed out, spine bowed and pass out. By that time she usually stopped breathing. The first time she did this, I got hysterical. This tiny child was lying on the floor unconscious, arms and legs positioned outward, and not breathing and I did not have a clue how to help her. Her only way of expressing anger or frustration resulted in a blue baby frequently needing help to remember how to breathe. This was the early seventies, and mouth to mouth resuscitation and CPR were relatively new procedures. Soon I was able to do it in my sleep. What, in any other child would have been a temper tantrum, was something altogether different in our house.

The first time this happened, I scooped her up and ran to the phone. As I was screaming at the emergency operator, Heather began to move. Thank God, she wasn't dead. I called John Tkach. I packed up both of my little girls and down the hill we raced. Heather checked out fine. She seemed not to have been bothered at all by these episodes, and there did not seem to have any lasting after effects, except on my wits and my nerves, I felt fifty years older.

I called Felicia again.

"Typical," she said, "get used to it and learn CPR quick. Usually," she added, "they rouse themselves, but if after 30 seconds or so she had not regained consciousness, get down on your hands and knees and breathe for her a few times. That should get her going."

I was startled into the reality that I was going to have to breathe for my daughter. This terrified me. It suddenly became apparent that the information I had read about concerning lack of perception of oxygen deprivation had a great deal more meaning than Dr. Crawford's admonition about not letting her fly in an unpressurized plane.

Once, the following year when we were visiting with Bruce's sister Esta, and her husband Bernie, Heather had a temper tantrum, and as my sister-in-law and her three girls watched in horror, she fell to the floor unconscious. When she had not resumed breathing spontaneously after about 30 seconds, I said to my nieces "Have you ever seen anyone do mouth to mouth?"

Esta was terrified as I got down on my hands and knees and breathed into Heather's mouth a few times until she came out of her seizure. When I was sure she was again breathing normally, I got up and walked away from her, as she sat up and composed herself.

My nieces stood there, mouths open, not knowing what was going on, while my sister in law, with hands shaking uncontrollably, poured herself a very large glass of wine.

Chapter Six

During the spring of that year, I learned there was a chapter of the Dysautonomia Foundation in Boston. I contacted them and attended several meetings. There were a handful of children in Massachusetts, and their mothers had banded together, with some dedicated friends to support one another, raise whatever funds they could for research and circulate information about the disease to Pediatricians, Obstetricians, and parents in the Jewish Community. One of the fund-raisers had been planned during that summer and I convinced Bruce we should take a chance, leave the girls with a baby-sitter, and drive to Newton for a Las Vegas Night.

When I walked into the hall, I said hellos and introduced Bruce to the people in the room whom I knew. I turned around and saw a young woman in a wheelchair. She was leaning to one side and was having great difficulty talking and moving. I felt the color drain out of my face, as I realized that this poor young woman, was one of the children who had survived into adolescence. My hands started to shake, my knees felt like they were made of rubber and I got that hot/cold sick/dizzy feeling you get when you are sure you are going to pass out. This was one thing for which I was not prepared. In front of me, was the vision of my worst personal nightmare. This was what I had convinced myself could never happen to my beautiful daughter, because we were the ones who were going to beat this thing and we were the ones who were going to make it. When we did, we were going to have a semi-healthy, normal child.

I had to get out of there, immediately. I could not bear to be in that room another minute. I thought if I stayed in that room, in her presence I would start screaming and never be able to stop. It had never occurred to me that the kinds of ravages this disease brought would result in an adult endpoint. I had never taken this disease to any kind of conclusion that did not have a happy ending. I really believed someone would come up with a cure. I positively believed someone would come up with a treatment that would let my child be healthy. At the absolute worst, at least she would survive it and Heather would be the one who would beat it. I could not allow myself to look at reality, open my eyes and embrace it.

Things were going relatively peacefully, we were adjusting to a life that had no blueprint. I was learning to think on my feet better. Bruce was becoming used to working all day, and then waking up for the midnight hospital runs, and Alyssa told most of her friends that "My sister is a hand-icapped little girl," in her most maternal tones.

There were some things that were definitely out of the norm. It was not until Heather was five months old that she responded to me as her mother. Until that time, she had no real preference for who was taking care of her. She did not smile until that time. She did not turn over until at least five months, and she did not crawl until almost ten months. Her attempts at speech were an unintelligible babble. Alyssa had been such a verbal toddler that trying to adjust to what Heather was trying to communicate was frustrating. If she was trying to say mama or dada, you only knew it because of the repetition and pointing. It became clear she was going to need intensive speech therapy. It was explained to me that she had no perception of where her tongue was in her mouth and no aware-ness of any of the other phenomenon that was required to produce intelligible speech. Even at age five, unless you knew what she was trying to say and was familiar with her syntax, you would have no clue as to what this child was talking about. Although all sorts of gross and fine motor development were a problem, speech was the biggest.

During that first year, I had become used to the strange things that happened. Stranger still, was the fact both Bruce and I had come to view any part of this as normal life. We had both been raised in typical 1950's and 60's households, and never had the opportunity or need to cultivate the coping skills we had developed in such a relatively short period of time. Neither of us had ever dreamed we would be so abruptly thrust into upheaval on an almost daily basis. Stages of crisis developed. The first of these stages was another part of our day to day routine. We tried to address these minor crises as a part of the business of living. While most mothers I knew carried Band-Aids in their purses for minor cuts and scrapes, I carried packages of alcohol prep pads and Steristrips to close lacerations until I could get them sutured.

Chapter Seven

In December of 1972, Heather was in the hospital with still another pneumonia. She was on her way to clearing her lungs, and this hospitalization was coming along fairly well. So well, in fact, I felt comfortable enough to go home one night to shower and sleep in my own bed.

When I arrived at the hospital at seven the next morning to feed Heather her breakfast, I was horrified when I looked at her eyes. They were completely gray and dull. I started to swear and scream. What had they done to my baby? I had stayed day and night for ten days so this would not happen, and the one time I left for seven hours, they had almost blinded her.

They tried to explain that the night nurse did not realize Heather had awakened when another child was being medicated. Heather must have rubbed her eyes across the sheet to do this kind of damage. She had to have dislodged her saran wrap patches and in so doing abraded her corneas. The nurse had not even checked on her to replace the patches or put drops in. It was useless to try to explain what had happened. In a rage I grabbed Heather, wrapped her in a blanket and raced home.

When I got her home, I called the ophthalmologist and explained the situation. He told me what to do, and said he would be available day and night if I needed him.

Her eyes looked lousy, and I worked on them twenty-four hours a day. Every three minutes, round the clock, I put her drops in. The ointments went in eight times a day trying to prevent infections.

The first Sunday morning in January, Heather woke up screaming. She could not open her eyes. I called Glenn Meltzer, our local ophthalmologist, and down we went to his office. After twenty minutes of bathing her eyelids in warm boric acid solution and carefully working on her lids, he got her eyes open. They looked as though someone had pared them out using a grapefruit spoon. The corneas were so badly abraded they defied an adequate description. Glenn called Mass Eye and Ear Infirmary in Boston, told us to get in the car and go.

They were waiting for us in the emergency entrance and immediately admitted Heather. We were met by Dr. Sumner Liebman, who explained our options to us. They were limited. Either tape her eyelids shut to facilitate healing, or sew her eyelids shut. I held Heather in my arms and talked to her softly, while the nurses put her tiny arms into restraints, put tincture of benzoin on her cheeks and forehead to make them more sticky, and taped both of her eyes shut. I could not leave her side for a minute. She was terrified, hysterical, blind and incapacitated by the arm restraints. They shot her full of antibiotics and tranquilizers to calm her down and prevent any further crisis, and we hoped for the best.

Bruce checked me into the Holiday Inn across the street from Mass General. That night we had a horrible ice storm. It took Bruce three hours to get home to Alyssa. Luckily, I had recently arranged with a student from the Anna Maria College, which was right around the corner from our house, to come over after her classes to be with Alyssa. Marge Hornyak and boyfriend Jerry Russell just about moved in for ten days to care for Alyssa. When Marge had late afternoon or evening classes, Jerry stayed. By the time Bruce got home from work, Lyssa was bathed, fed and ready to cuddle up with her dad for an hour or two before bed. They were lifesavers.

It snowed or sleeted every day that week in January 1974. Each day was worse than the one that had preceded it. Every day I would promise Heather the tapes would come off soon, and every time they took them off to reevaluate her eyes, there was no improvement. I remember the Sunday morning of the following week when I called my mother in New Jersey. She told me that since everything here was so terrible, she did not want to give me any more bad news. So she had not told me that my dear, dear grandfather, at 96, had taken ill. He had died earlier that morning. I sat down on the floor of the phone booth and cried. Cried for my grandfather, cried for both my daughters, cried for my husband, cried for myself.

I paced the floor, sat in Heather's room then paced some more. When I was sure Heather was asleep, I went down to the first floor of the hospital, found the tunnel to the General, and went to the Blood Bank. Since there was nothing I could do for anyone I loved, I felt helpless. Maybe I could give blood, and help someone I did not know. They looked at me and told me to get on the scale. They then informed me that to donate blood, I would have to weigh at least 115 pounds. I begged them. Please make an exception. Maybe, if I weighed 112. But 101 pounds was definitely out. Now I not only felt helpless, I felt useless.

One day during that week, Marge and Jerry brought Alyssa into Boston. This was the only part of that week that appeared even faintly normal. I ate three meals a day in the Mass General cafeteria, and if there was a better way to lose weight, I had yet to find it. Every day was the same, I would talk to Heather, read to her and try to play with a two and a half year old child whose eyes were taped shut, and had both arms in restraints. It always amazed me that she was able to take as much as she did and still be a smiling child. The rest of those days were all the same, when she slept, I would eat, and at night I would go back to the Holiday Inn, take a bath, take ten of Valium, and try to sleep. Most nights I slept two or three hours at best and would walk back to the hospital at five or six a.m. I had called one of the women's clothing distributors in town and told them I was going to take a cab over to 75 Kneeland St. and pick up some clothing for myself. Since Bruce was in women's clothing business, all of the houses knew me, knew my sizes and preferences. They were great, and had skirts, slacks, sweaters and blouses set aside. I did not bother to try them on, just signed the invoices, and left. There was a small shopping area near the hotel where I got some shoes as all I had with me were the heavy snow boots that I had worn the first day we came to Boston, and I even a found a place that had some decent underwear. As far as other grooming materials were concerned, all I had were the basics I had purchased at the hotel gift shop. Most of the time I was relatively put together. After twelve days they let me take Heather home.

Chapter Eight

When we got her settled back at the house, she acclimated very well. She found if she crawled around the house backward, she could get just about everywhere. Naturally, we put gates at the steps and in front of the kitchen, but all else was navigable. The only time she really screamed was when she was totally frustrated by the gates.

Although, I cannot remember exactly how many months we had to live with those tapes on Heather's face. I could never forget what her cheeks looked like after the countless applications of tincture of benzoin and adhesive tape closures finally came off. Her face was vaguely reminiscent of raw hamburger on a plate. Each time one of the tapes came off for an application of medication or a progress check a little more skin ripped away.

When the tapes came off for the last time, there were scars on both corneas. Looking through those scars must have been like looking through badly smudged glass. There was no way to adequately describe what her cheeks and forehead looked like. Every time I saw those cheeks and visible scars in her eyes, my stomach did a 180.

During that time, Heather developed some strange eating habits. I felt obliged to indulge them. Another oddity of this disease seemed to be the way her body metabolized food. She could eat her own weight in food every five or six days. In other words, she ate like a pig, but grew and gained very poorly. Since she could not taste the food she ate, she only ate foods that appealed to her on other levels. She liked red food, but would not touch anything green. She liked food with strong smells. It would not be unusual to see her eat a peeled onion the way other children would eat an apple. Her all time favorite food was French apple pie. It not only looked great, it smelled wonderful.

Bruce would go on regular buying trips to New York City, and the owner of Kenny's Steak House always sent him home with a restaurant-sized French apple pie and a cheesecake for Heather. Once when we had been in Manhattan for a check up at NYU, we were at Kenny's for dinner. Kenny was utterly charmed by both girls and floored by the quantity of French apple pie Heather packed away. Every time Kenny saw Bruce, he asked about the girls and boxed pies for Heather and Alyssa. If she were lucky, Lyssa would get a taste of the cheesecake, but she to be quick. Heather could usually manage to finish them both off in less than a week.

For snacking, Heather liked the Gerber junior spaghetti and meatballs, because it was her favorite shade of red. In addition to her regular meals, she would eat seven junior sized jars of this flavor every day. I remember being in the supermarket, buying my 49 jars of this junior spaghetti and meatballs for the week, and being asked how many days it would take my twins to eat that much spaghetti. Some days it was just too much trouble to explain, and I answered about three weeks.

Heather loved lox, eggs and onions. Whenever she was in the hospital and able to eat solid food, my father-in-law's best friend, Jack Pearl, would come up every Sunday morning with a huge platter of lox, eggs and onions, bagels with cream cheese and lox, fried potatoes and kippers for Heather's breakfast. I don't remember ever asking Jack to bring Heather her breakfast, but he knew she loved it, and it simply arrived Sunday mornings at 9 a.m. She had an unusual effect on people. She always brought out the best in them. The dietary staff must have thought it a little out of the ordinary, but every menu I had to fill out for Heather generally had least two color coordinated entrees and two desserts, sometimes, three.

Chapter Nine

During the months that it took for Heather's eyes to return to semi-normal, we went to her ophthalmologist in Boston at least once a week. Most of our local doctors signed off when they realized they were in over their heads.

On one awful trip to Boston, I took Heather to Dr. Liebman, and he suggested that we give serious consideration to sewing her eyelids shut during such visual crises. This was not one of the options I wanted to hear. On the way home, about 2:30 in the afternoon, I realized I had not eaten since seven that morning, and even though I was not hungry, I should eat. Heather had not eaten in an hour or so and was howling for something red. We stopped at a truck stop in Westboro called Harry's. I ordered some spaghetti for Heather and a hot roast beef sandwich for myself. Still very distracted and upset by what I heard from Dr. Liebman, and not paying a great deal of attention to what I was eating, I choked. Until that time I had never realized when you are choking, it is impossible to utter a single sound. I wanted to scream, but nothing came out. Heather just looked at me strangely. There was no one sitting near us, and the thought crossed my mind that I was going to die in Harry's and be found face down in my mashed potatoes and gravy. I grabbed my plate and smashed it on the floor before I passed out.

The next thing I remembered was hanging upside down being held by an enormous truck driver. He was slapping me on the back, hard. These were the pre Heimlich days. When I came around, he put me down and finished his lunch. I never found out his name.

It took well over a year for Heather to master the coordination necessary to walk. For her it was not a matter of reflex behavior. She had to be taught all of the components of walking. She also had to learn to break her falls by putting her arms out in front of her. I do not think I had fully realized the danger inherent in not being able to perceive pain. Since she had become mobile, she put herself in line for a whole new set of dangers. One Saturday morning, I was in the kind of semi sleep that I allowed myself in quieter times. Heather was so conditioned to her eye drops, and Alyssa was so programmed to the timer, that when Heather woke up, frequently she would walk over to me in bed and I would put her drops in while half asleep. Alyssa set the timer for every ten minutes and it was a workable situation. On that particular morning, Heather had been up for about a half an hour and she and Alyssa were watching cartoons. Bruce and I were still in our semi conscious states, when Heather and Alyssa came into the bedroom and I immediately sprung to full attention. There was a gash in Heather's forehead about an inch and a half long and a full quarter inch wide. She had fallen against the television and hit her head on the part of the door that projected out to allow access to the control knobs. She did not cry or seem terribly bothered by the cut, but the blood was running into her eyes and it was making it difficult to watch Scooby Doo. Alyssa realized there was a problem and wanted me to get a Band-Aid for her to put on Heather's forehead.

That cut took 8 stitched to close and was the first of countless trips to the emergency room for facial lacerations. She never did seem to get the hang of putting out her arms to break her falls, and after a while her forehead looked like a roadmap of the Northeast Interstate System.

In the bigger picture, this was one of the least of our problems. Most of the time, it was no more than an inconvenience.

Chapter Ten

In June of 1973 Heather got sick. I was used to the drill by this time and I called John Tkach, told him that I was going to admit her directly and asked him to call Hahnemann Hospital and give admitting orders. She was admitted with aspiration pneumonia, her usual diagnosis. I got her organized, said hello to all of the staff that was on the three to eleven shift, and prepared myself for the usual, customary rituals. Those included making sure I had a couple packs of cigarettes and a place to grab an occasional nap, or shower, the usuals.

I had begun to feel cocky. It did not appear that this was anything out of the ordinary as far as pneumonia admissions went. I was beginning to think of myself as a paramedic/wonderwoman/super mother. I could, after all, pass a naso-gastric tube, or a rectal tube, suction, perform I.P.P.B. treatments, do postural drainage and percussion, give injections, do CPR, check blood pressure and pulse, the usual. Temperature by touch, was my specialty. I could put my hand on Heather's belly and get a temperature accurate to within .2 of a degree. I had lulled myself into a genuine false sense of security. I had also begun to believe that there really was a way we could beat this thing for sure.

However, things were beginning to deteriorate. Heather was not responding to the drugs and treatments. Her temperature was not coming down, her lungs were not clearing and her behavior was becoming quite erratic. Her cheerful demeanor was gone, as she was getting sicker and harder to deal with, not only on the medical level, but the psychological as well.

About a week into this admission, John Tkach came to me and told me he was uncomfortable having Heather in Hahnemann. They did not have a pediatric ICU and he wanted her in St. Vincent's Hospital, across town. He said that there would always be a Pedi house officer available and that they were far better prepared for crisis management. It honestly had never occurred to me that Hahnemann was not well prepared. I had never dreamed that she could get into a major life-threatening crisis, and on that day in June, I was totally unprepared to even conceive of the kinds of danger she could experience. I was still blissfully ignorant. My higher education was about to commence.

Chapter Eleven

We packed Heather into an ambulance and Bruce followed us across the city of Worcester to St. Vincent's Hospital on the East Side of the city. They admitted her directly into a private room on the seventh floor, as they wanted to isolate and observe, thinking that she might have had an infection that had yet to be diagnosed. They implemented sterile procedures, and we had to gown, glove and mask before entering the room. Her temperature was dangerously high and there were two IV lines in place to give her fluids. Heather's face was flushed and she was crying irregularly and gulping air between breaths. She was wired with a cardiac monitor, and was to have around the clock nurses to watch her.

Before the resident had a chance to start his workup, she arrested. There are no words to describe the terror and anguish I felt standing next to my daughter's crib when her heart stopped.

The nurse on duty with Heather, Celeste, ordered Bruce to open the door and scream, "CODE BLUE ROOM 724." She ripped off her mask, climbed into the crib and started to do mouth to mouth. I ripped off my mask, climbed into the crib and started to do closed cardiac massage. I did not think about what I was doing or what I was feeling, I did what had to be done. Within thirty seconds the tiny, single crib room filled with nurses, doctors, respiratory therapists and lab people falling all over each other. A priest was ready for last rites as St. Vincent's was a Catholic hospital and this was standard operating procedure for all CODE BLUE announcements.

Celeste and I had resuscitated her by the time everyone else arrived and Bruce and I were asked to leave. I resisted, but knew if I turned myself into a pain in the ass, I would be systematically excluded in less critical times. If one was not part of the solution, one was very definitely part of the problem, and they had enough problems to deal with at that time.

The orderlies planted two chairs by the door, and that was where Bruce and I sat and waited. There was a nun by my side, and a priest at the door. A social worker, named Katy Prior magically appeared and gave me a cigarette, a big no-no for the nuns, but Katy whispered in my ear something to the effect that if the nuns did not like it, they could go and screw themselves. I actually laughed, rather hysterically, but a laugh nonetheless, as I conjured a mental image of a nun doing that. Katy got us coffee and called our friends to pick up Alyssa from nursery school and take care of her. She asked them to try to prepare her for all of the possible eventualities as best they could, and then Katy called the rest of the family. The network of social services was preparing us for the possible forthcoming death of our daughter and they wanted the support system in place. That was the first time this was done. Katy and I formed an immediate bond. She had a way of cutting through all of the bullshit and getting down to the specifics of what needed to be done.

One of the residents came out and told us he thought that Heather was bleeding into her intestinal cavity. He suspected this because her belly was extremely distended. Logically, he thought, there must be an accumulation of blood in her abdomen. Not one person in that hospital had ever seen or read about Familial Dysautonomia and none of them had a clue about the strange and bizarre nature of the things that Heather's body did. He wanted permission to perform a four-quadrant abdominal tap to ascertain the location of the bleed. This, he explained, would entail inserting a needle into her abdomen at four spots to isolate the area of the bleeding. I refused. He looked at me as if I was crazy and started to treat me like an idiotic, hysterical mother. Taking a deep breath, I looked at him and explained to him that one of the weirder things about my child was that when she was upset she gulped tremendous quantities of air between cries. I told him that if her stomach was not flat in thirty minutes, I would give permission for his tap. He told me again that he was not sure he had that kind of time because she was bleeding, and that I was crazy and demanded that I give permission. I refused and shot Bruce a look that said, "Please listen to me and not him." Bruce also refused.

The resident was furious and swearing as he reentered the room. He came out twenty minutes later and told me that her belly was flat and the room smelled terrible. As I started to smile, she coded again.

Her temp had shot up to 107 degrees, and they were unable to get it down. They resuscitated her again, packed her armpits and groin in ice and put her on a cooling blanket. When she finally stabilized, they moved her down the hall to the Pedi ICU. The situation was extremely critical.

John Tkach arrived and we placed a conference call to Felicia Axelrod in New York City. John always included me in conference calls because he realized there were things I noticed that he might not. As I said before, his gift truly was in his gentle intelligence and sensitivity, not ego. When he listened, he heard. Not many people do that.

Chapter Twelve

One of Felicia's many useful suggestions were that I sit down with every new shift of house staff and introduce them to Heather's case. The interns, residents, nurses, respiratory therapists, dietitians, anyone who can into contact with Heather, had to be carefully briefed about Dysautonomia, taking particular care to elaborate on the very extraordinary and subtle nuances of the disease. There was not one person in that hospital that had ever read about it in their medical training and simple omissions because of ignorance could be life threatening. This briefing policy became standard procedure every time Heather was admitted. House staff would congregate in the seventh floor conference room. I would talk. They would listen. There was generally one intern or resident who strode into the room with lots of attitude. He or she more often than not lost it and a whole lot of arrogance before he or she left the one of the briefings.

It truly was an unusual thing to see doctors willingly cater to a parent regarding treatment or a judgment call. It was a frequently painful responsibility I neither enjoyed nor ignored.

This first admission to St. Vincent's was a learning experience for all of us. Heather had symptoms and swings in her vital signs that seemed to be impossible for humans to survive. She would spike a temperature of 106 one minute, and twenty minutes later, she would bottom out at 95. We would alternately pack her in ice, then throw off the ice bags and put her under heated blanket. Her blood pressure was never the same twice and vacillated between hyper and hypotension hourly. When I held these strange briefings, I would see looks of disbelief and could hear people muttering under their breaths that I had to be either exaggerating or certifiably insane. After the first week residents were coming to me with questions and asking for advice on treatments. This power switch was frightening and the responsibility, staggering.

During those first weeks at St. V's, I got to know all of the nurses and house doctors in each rotation assigned to pediatrics. I knew whom I liked, whom I trusted, and more importantly, those whom I did not want coming anywhere near my child. I called the chief of the unit, Noel Bontempo, whenever there were disputes to be mediated, and had the head of respiratory therapy, Andre, bring me a carton of cigarettes every other day. Never leaving, I slept either in a chair in the unit, on a couch in the lounge, or when I got lucky an empty bed on the floor. Friends turned into stand-in parents for Alyssa, and did a phenomenal job of keeping her together body and soul. I thanked God for them daily. Bruce came in before opening the store in the morning, afternoons at lunch and for supper after he closed the store. We did so enjoy the cuisine of the Chez St. V's cafeteria. Carl and Sylvia brought up clean clothes, snacks, cosmetics, shampoo and everything else I needed. I showered in the floor showers, and spent almost three consecutive weeks there, before I felt comfortable enough to go home and sleep in my own bed between midnight and six a.m. Exhaustion was constant, and migraine headaches were a frequent problem. It was not unusual to see me sitting in a chair in the unit with my head lying on the windowsill, balancing a rubber glove full of crushed ice on the side of my head.

Heather was in the pediatric Intensive Care Unit of St. Vincent's almost all summer. When she finally came home, she managed to stay home almost four whole weeks until her next admission.

The visits to St.V.'s were becoming commonplace. I would admit her directly into the unit and there we would stay for however many weeks it took for the pneumonia to resolve. The pediatric nurses were becoming like sisters to me and the interns and residents were my classmates. We spent months learning together how to keep Heather alive, when her body was in armed rebellion against itself.

Our home now had a suction machine, an intermittent positive pressure machine for breathing exercises and the administration of inhaled bronchiodilators, oxygen tanks, syringes, padded tongue blades for seizures, butterfly closures, Shirmer papers for testing eye moisture, liter sized bottles of saline and pint bottles of methyl cellulose for her daily eye care, industrial sized tubes of Ilotycin ophthalmic ointment, splints, braces, restraints, different antibiotics, Valium and Thorazine. It was not unusual to get calls late at night from one of our doctors or the town pharmacist to ask if we had a particular drug in our personal stock.

Everyone in contact with Heather knew her daily routine of drops, pulmonary therapy of percussion and postural drainage, suctioning and I.P.P.B. breathing treatments and the endless meds.

Heather was among very rare group of children. There were less than three hundred documented cases, and we felt obliged to do whatever anyone asked to try to find a treatment or cure. Since there was such a small patient base from which to draw, we had to accede to what we felt were reasonable requests from researchers, regardless of the need or the physical discomfort. When the Massachusetts Eye and Ear Infirmary wanted some conjunctival tissue to calculate the number of goblet cells in the membranes surrounding Heather's eyes, we went to Mass Eye and Ear and let them remove some tissue from the conjunctiva of her eye. When NYU wanted a piece of sural nerve tissue for an experiment they were running, we went to New York and allowed them to cut into Heather's leg and take a piece of nerve tissue to perform a sural nerve biopsy. Had we known how large of an incision was needed to remove the nerve segment, we would have probably thought twice before giving permission. Both Bruce and I were more than a little surprised and appalled to see an almost two inch long incision on the back of the calf of Heather's left leg. We had been under the impression that it was a much smaller procedure. When Yale New Haven Medical wanted skin from Bruce and me for genetic analysis, we went to a surgeon and had pieces of skin cut out of our right forearms, had them packed in dry ice and shipped to New Haven. It seemed everyone wanted blood and consequently there were frozen vials of our blood sent to whoever needed it to look for a carrier test. Bits and pieces of us were all over the country with very few practical and useable results. What they did find out was that almost 90 percent of all of Heather's unmyelinated nerve cells were undeveloped. The unmyelinated cells produce a neurochemical necessary for nerve impulses to bridge the neural synapse. Her neural synapses were like a bridge with the middle section missing. There was no way to make the connection and bridge the gap. That accounted for the lack of response from her autonomic and central nervous systems. This disease was a nightmare from hell, and we felt like narcoleptics.

Chapter Thirteen

Eventually we found that we were able to work ourselves in a state that passed for normalcy and a tolerable rhythm. We realized something had to be done in regard to speech and physical therapy. In the middle 1970s Massachusetts passed the Chapter 766 Education Act insuring that all handicapped children between the ages of three and twenty-one receive appropriate education at the expense of the state. We enrolled Heather in the Worcester State College Collaborative Preschool. It was designed specifically for severely speech-disabled children. With that, along with one-on-one speech therapy sessions held three times a week, formal education commenced when Heather was about three.

In order to insure her relative health and safety, Heather was always to be accompanied by a private duty nurse when she went to school. I was not at all comfortable with the idea of a stranger watching my very unique child, but more than happy for the four hours of free time, three times a week. I suggested the Special Education administrator interview and hire Sharon Luftig, a dear friend who was also a registered nurse. Sharon knew Heather almost as well as I did, and did double duty as Alyssa's stand-in mother. There were countless times that we had called Sharon and her husband Ron, a Ph.D. and researcher at the Worcester Foundation for Experimental Biology, in the middle of the night and told them that we were bringing Alyssa over on our way to St. Vincent's Hospital. Alyssa spent weeks at a time at the Luftig house. Gillian, their youngest daughter, was Alyssa's best friend, Miriam and Aimee were the older sisters that Lyssa never had, and Sharon and Ron were often the parents who soothed our daughter's tears in out absence.

Sharon was delighted to act as Heather's nurse. Her children were all in school and it was an ideal part time job for her. Sharon would arrive at our house just before the school bus, and she and Heather would go to school together. Sharon was very sensitive to the subtle nuances and signals that often served as Heather's early warning system. Often when they came home from preschool, Sharon would tell me to be alert for an impending pneumonia.

Before the Commonwealth of Massachusetts could certify Heather as a special needs student, they required documentation. It was easy enough to document the physical problems, but it became necessary to try to administer an IQ test for proper evaluation. The staff psychologist for our school union performed this. We set a date and decided the easiest way to conduct this examination was to hold it at the Paxton Center School.

Off we went to school one morning to meet with the school psychologist. I completed the necessary paperwork and the actual testing commenced. About twenty minutes into it, Heather started to fall asleep at her desk. She did not appear to be ill, just tired. I suggested to the examiner that she might do better if I got her some cold black coffee. The look that crossed that man's face was worth the price of admission. Finding the school cafeteria, I got her a cup of strong black coffee, cooled it with ice and gave it to Heather to drink. I could just imagine the report about the bizarre little girl who liked her coffee strong, black and cold. The coffee had little effect. It seemed to me something was about to happen medically, and I tried to explain this to the examiner. He said, there would be no problem and he would be happy to reschedule. With that assurance, we left.

Two hours later, we were in the Pedi ICU with aspiration pneumonia. Accidentally, several months later, I saw a copy of the initial report: the one that was supposed to have been invalidated. The conclusion was that not only was Heather physically handicapped, but mentally challenged as well.

They had estimated her IQ at 70. I went ballistic. They had not listened to anything they had been told concerning the nature of the disease. I threatened to sue the Department of Education and name the examiner as incompetent and not up to the job required of him. I think I threatened to sue at least half of the special education staff. Finally it was agreed that all copies of the original report would be destroyed in my presence and new testing would be done at Worcester State College using examiners who had made themselves familiar with the literature about the learning disabilities associated with Familial Dysautonomia. Roughly three months later, after Heather had started at the Collaborative Preschool, she was re-evaluated. Her IQ measured at 120. I had never believed that my daughter had a future as a nuclear physicist or brain surgeon, but I had never doubted that considering the constraints of her body, she performed incredibly well. Her ability to adapt to the mislocations of her body demonstrated her more than adequate potential to learn, and apply information.

Chapter Fourteen

One night I went to a Dysautonomia meeting and Bruce was in charge of getting the girls into bed. When I got home around 11 p.m., he said everything was fine. I kissed both girls and went to bed. When I got up the next morning to get the kids ready for school and when I got Heather out of her bunny sleeper I was horrified when I saw her left foot. It was bluish purple and swollen roughly twice its normal size. What had happened?

It seemed the night before Heather was playing supermarket in the lower kitchen cabinets when a can of green beans fell out of the lazy Susan cupboard and landed on her foot. Bruce thought nothing of it because Heather was playing happily with her puzzles after and later went to bed without any problems.

This time I called U Mass Med. Center, where her orthopedist was and announced that I was bringing her in immediately. For the previous eighteen months, Heather had been seeing Dr. Arthur Pappas as she had severe back and shoulder spasms and had also developed significant scoliosis or spinal curvature. Dr. Pappas's practice has always been exclusive to children and professional athletes. Since we had met him when he first was called in to consult when one of Heather's shoulders had frozen in a muscle spasm, he had always gone out of his way to accommodate her unusual problems with gentle, caring precision and expertise.

Dr. Pappas took one look at her foot and ordered immediate x-rays. There was no question in either of our minds that her foot was broken, it was only a matter of how badly. Luckily it was not a displaced fracture, and since she was having neither pain nor difficulty walking, we decided not to put a cast on it. We agreed a cast could pose even more of a threat than the unset fracture, as there would be no way of knowing if there were any circulatory problems because of Heather's inability to perceive the pain or pressure. As impossible as it seemed, Heather was completely oblivious to the metatarsal fracture that would have had any normal child shrieking in pain.

Although Heather did not perceive pain, she did acknowledge uncomfortable feelings. She hated to have her hair combed or brushed. She screamed like she was being tortured when I had to comb her hair out after it was shampooed. Some of her systems underfunctioned, while others overfunctioned. Touching her head with a comb or brush was agony, but bone fractures were not. Another strange manifestation was although she produced almost no moisture in her eyes, she produced copious amounts of saliva and stomach acid. She drooled constantly as she had trouble swallowing the saliva. There was too much of one thing and not nearly enough of another.

At about three and a half, Heather's eyes deteriorated again. Although they had never been very good, this promised to be a horror show. I called New York. Dr. Axelrod told me they had just begun to experiment with a new device; soft contact lenses were used as bandages over corneal ulcerations. We told her to set up the appointment immediately we were on our way.

The next day we saw Dr. Robert D'Amico, chief of Ophthalmology at St. Vincent's Hospital in New York City. He fitted Heather with soft lenses and told us we needed to keep them wet constantly and to put saline drops in her eyes as often as it was necessary to keep the lenses moist. We were to try to determine the frequency and go with it. He wanted to see Heather the next day and then again, one day later. We lost one lens the first day.

We went across the river and stayed with my mother, Minna, in her apartment in New Jersey and traveled back and forth to Manhattan from there. The second night my father-in-law called. Our house had been burglarized. The Paxton police chief had called him and he in turn, called us. The burglars had taken everything in the living room, but the couch. The television was gone, the stereo and the paintings off the wall. Also they had taken the vacuum cleaner, my jewelry and the sterling silver that Bruce's grandmother had given us when we got married. What did we want them to do Carl had asked? All we could think of to tell them to do was to board up the broken door and window and ask the police to look for our things.

When we returned from New York City a few days later with bottles of soft lenses and both kids in tow, we walked into an empty living room I felt violated and abused. It made me physically ill to know that someone had rifled through my underwear and rummaged through everything we owned looking for goods to fence. What could we do other than call the insurance company? Bruce was philosophical and calm. These were, after all, only things. They had to compensate us for the stolen property, and wherever possible, we tried to replace the lost items, but the peace of mind concerning the sanctity of our home could never be replaced.

The schedule for Heather's drops was set at every six minutes, and at that we were losing lenses at the rate of about one every three days. We were not wealthy and were just managing with all of the doctor's bills and prescriptions costs and had to find a way to deal with this new expense. We'd paid the $100 to replace each lost lens. We would shrug our collective shoulders in frustration. When you live in a state of shocked flux, you lose the ability to perceive problems clearly. The analogy of not being able to see the forest for the trees comes to mind. We had to deal with the immediate problems, frequently becoming unable to cope with the larger ones. At $100 per lens replacement, sometimes as many as a dozen or so a month, it quickly added up.

During this time, my mother had come up for a visit, and when she saw what was happening to us, she took it upon herself to write to Bausch and Lomb and tell them about our unique problem. They wrote back about a week later and told us that for as long as we needed them, the lenses would be delivered to us free of charge. Thank god for mother's without terminal tunnel vision.

Chapter Fifteen

Not all of our experiences were critical. There were some that were, frankly, a riot. During the summer of 1973 we decided that we really needed a vacation. We rented a house in Bass River on Cape Cod for ten days. We packed everything, including a baby sitter to spell us when Heather was napping. The Cape was lovely and the vacation sorely needed.

The trip home was a traffic nightmare. It took us almost eight hours to drive 80 miles home. Every ten minutes or less, someone was asking are we home yet.

As we finally got off the Bourne Bridge, Bruce announced that the next day he was hiring someone to put a pool in the backyard. After that hellish drive from the Cape, he met with no resistance. The very next day, we hired a contractor and ordered a pool built. We figured that two vacations like the one we had just had, would more than pay for the cost of the pool. We just forgot about what it would cost to have a deck built around it, and an eight-foot high stockade fence containing the entire area.

Construction began almost immediately. The first thing the contractor did was dig an enormous hole; right in the middle of the leach field for our septic system. Eventually, by the following summer, we had our pool. Heather hated it. Gratefully she hated being anywhere near the water. She hated to be bathed, and she screamed every time anyone even suggested a shower. So keeping her away from the pool was not a problem. But she was a very curious and ravenous child.

By that time she was eating me out of house and home. She was three ears old, weighed about 25 pounds and ate like a body builder. Her appetite was insatiable and her intake, unbelievable.

One Sunday we had company for the afternoon. We spent a very pleasant day eating, swimming and drinking wine. All of the kids were playing or swimming and all of the adults were relaxing. Heather was happily going from my lap to Bruce's and generally enjoying herself as well. She was having such a good time that no one noticed she was toddling from person to person quietly sipping white wine from everyone's glasses. When I went to bring her into the house for supper and her bath, I found her sitting propped up next to a chair, giggling madly and drunk.

She was so plastered she couldn't stand up without falling down. She was having a great time and feeling even less pain than usual. It took three hours and two pots of strong, cold black coffee for her to sober up.

There was one afternoon I can remember being hung up in bumper to bumper traffic on Route 9 in Shrewsbury. I had gone to pick up an air filtration machine someone thought would help Heather's breathing during the night. I always felt duty bound to try almost anything one of her doctors suggested that might make the nights easier and this of course, sounded fairly logical. The traffic was awful and the kids were miserable and complaining. By the time I had gotten home. I had pretty much forgotten about the details of the trip. Alyssa, it seems, had not.

Two or three days later, I got a call from Alyssa's first grade teacher. She was concerned about a story Alyssa had written down. She thought it was marginally inappropriate for a six-year old. As she told me, her concerns were about Alyssa's use of proper language in her classroom. She said she would send me a copy of the story and would I please take the correct measures. The story went something like this: "One day we were stuck in traffic. I was hungry and my sister to go to the bathroom. My mother said,

"I wish this dumb son of a bitch would move his ass." I said 'I wish the dumb son of a bitch would move his ass, too.' My mother said "Alyssa!!!'"

I thought her use of language was completely correct and only a little inappropriate.

One winter when we were having a ferocious Nor'easter. Snow was blowing into our attic through the ventilation louvers. None of us knew this until late that evening, when we were getting ready for bed. Bruce was in the shower, and I was reading in bed when I noticed that water was dripping down on the bed through the ceiling light fixture. We pulled down the ladder that led to the attic and found it full of snow. In tandem, Bruce loaded the snow into an old laundry basket and handed it down the ladder to me, and I then ran outside, dumped it out and then gave him the basket to fill again. After two hours of this back breaking exercise most of the snow was cleared except for a small amount deep in the outer edges of the rafters. At that point, I had had enough and was exhausted and went back to my reading in bed.

Compulsive could be Bruce's middle name and he just had to get that last little bit of snow out of the attic. While trying to balance on the cross-beam and reach out to the farthest point of the edge of the attic, his foot slipped off the rafter.

Lying in bed, I roared with laughter as this three foot long leg, with boot attached at the foot, crashed through the ceiling above my head. Howling with vast amusement and exhaustion, I thought it was just about the funniest thing I had ever seen. Bruce did not unequivocally agree. He was howling also, but at me. Didn't I have any idea how much this little disaster of his was going to cost to repair? He totally failed to see any humor in this occurrence. Although he was furious, I could not stop laughing. I tried to explain how comical this looked, but he was not amused. He was in no mood to take the joke. He saw only dollar signs to fix the ceiling, while I saw the funniest thing I had seen in years. A couple of years after that, I bought him a T-shirt that had the word COMPUL-SIVE on the front, with every vertical line in the word dotted.

Chapter Sixteen

As I have previously mentioned, not all of Heather's doctors were what she needed. When she was an infant she was seen regularly at the Cornea Clinic at Mass Eye and Ear Infirmary in Boston. Her doctor was the chief of Cornea service at the time. A very important man, or so we were led to believe.

There was a winter day we went into Boston for an appointment. Heather had a corneal ulceration in one of her eyes and I was afraid that it was beginning to infect. After waiting in the ancient and cavernous waiting room for the "DOCTOR" we were foisted off to an intern. I packed up the snowsuits, the diaper bag, the bottles, jars of baby food and all of the other stuff that accompanied the visit and schlepped all of it and both of my daughters in to see the "DOCTOR."

This was shortly before I had abandoned the illusion that God was second only to doctors. This doctor was a peach fuzz faced intern on the ophthalmology rotation who looked like he had just biked over from Boston Latin High School. I was still naive and truly believed that if the "DOCTOR" had sent my daughter and her extremely unusual case to someone else, he at least had a working knowledge of her disease and the very tenuous condition of her eyes. This doctor/apprentice looked at her eyes and without consulting either her history in the chart or the great "DOC-

TOR", prescribed a tube of boric acid ointment for her eyes and sent us home.

I was still young and gullible not yet found the voice I needed to question everything and beat it to death until I understood the logic behind it. I took home the prescription and started to use it, and almost blinded my daughter in the bargain.

A week later, angry and frustrated, after the crisis had just barely been averted, I called my lawyer. This had to be malpractice on the part of the "DOCTOR". I was full of moral indignation and wrath and I wanted revenge. What I really wanted was to wish on the arrogant physician and his student, a portion of the pain, suffering and guilt we had endured and the near blindness with which Heather almost had to live. What I really wanted was blood.

The lawyer said he would look into it. This was the early 70s before the era of litigation for fun and profit. When he called back several days later, he told us that he had spoken to several ophthalmologists and there was no question in any of their minds this had been an incidence of negligence and malpractice. But not one of them was willing to testify against another doctor, no matter how blatant the misconduct. Their concern was in protecting their own backs.

One of the only regrets I have is that I have so few memories that do not involve major crises. I have almost no memories of any of Alyssa's accomplishments or milestones. I have lost almost all of the 70s. The only newsworthy event I remember at all is the Watergate hearings. I remember them, only because they were on television during one of Heather's hospitalizations and they droned nonstop on the television in the unit. The only song I remember from that time is "Bohemian Rhapsody" by Queen, and the only movie I can remember from that time is "Brian's Song." I can clearly remember being alone in the living room one night watching it and weeping uncontrollably. I know too, it must have been on in late November or December, because that was the only time of the year Bruce had to work late every night. In the retail business, it is a necessity, and this was often a time I used to feel particularly isolated and sorry for myself. This month of the retail calendar had always been my annual period of single-parenthood.

If one was to ask me who was the president was in 1975, I couldn't answer unless I looked it up. But ask me how to pass a rectal tube or suction bronchial tubes and I wouldn't skip a beat before giving a detailed explanation. My priority was one thing: Heather. I will be sorrow-filled to my dying day, because of my lack of knowledge and memory of my other daughter, and my lack of attention to her. I mourn the passing of her childhood from the ages of 2 to 7. I can never get that time back, or her personal history and milestones.

Chapter Seventeen

It seemed holidays were usually marked at St. Vincent's Hospital. There were Halloweens, Independence Days, Memorial Days, and Christmases that, for the most part, ran into one another. One fortunate Fourth of July, we were actually home and not in one of our many crises. In an attempt to show some gratitude for the staff at St. V.'s we had a pool party for all of the pediatric house staff. Remarkably, everyone who was not on duty came. The party lasted all day, and when the 7 am to 3 PM shift finished their workday, they came too. They had become the extended family we were missing. The only close family we had in the area was Carl and Sylvia. Locally, there were no aunts, uncles or cousins the girls could relate to, and the house staff at St. V's stood in. We knew about all of their families and they knew all about ours. I remember trying to console the Pedi head nurse, Cynthia, when her nephew was admitted for a possible broken neck. It was the only way to give back a little of the caring. I cried with Celeste when her marriage was breaking up. We had coffee together in the mornings, lunch and cigarettes breaks in the cafeteria in the late afternoons. Most of the cafeteria was dedicated to staff only and family and friends of the patients were not supposed to take tables there. But there was never a time that I ever sat in the family section. I was there so often and so long I was accepted as staff. I remember when Martha got engaged, and when Beth was dating and hopelessly in love.

I used to dread every July when a new group of interns and residents started pediatric rotation, and the thought of having to listen to them grumble and complain. There were so many changes of the house officers that came and went annually; our usual reliance was on the nursing staff. This was the one constant.

One Christmas, Heather was in St. V's and on the mend. One of the night nurses, Beth, decided that it would be fun for Heather to have a special Christmas, and when Bruce and I were downstairs eating, she decorated Heather like a Christmas tree. She hung tinsel all over her shoulders and on top of her hair, and scotch taped ornaments to her ears. It was, possibly, Heather's best Christmas. I know it is the only one that stands out in my memory. Heather paraded all over the ICU and up and down the hall of the seventh floor, dragging her IV pole behind her. Since it was also Chanukah that week, the following day we celebrated with candle lighting and potato latkes for all.

Chapter Eighteen

During the summer of 1972, Heather was in the hospital with a very tenacious pneumonia. It was a hot, miserable summer, and one night was particularly horrid. There was no air conditioning, and the temperature in Heather's room was hovering around the 90-degree mark. The fans only pushed around the oppressive humidity-laden air. Heather was dehydrating faster and faster and no one could hit a vein for the IV that she needed. They would come in and stick her and stick her. Even though she could not feel the needles going into her, she hated having to be restrained for the procedure. For hours, each of the nurses and phlebotomists tried, with no success. John Tkach came in for evening rounds. He appeared to be just as miserable and sweaty as everyone else in the building. He went into Heather's room determined to start the IV. After more than an hour of trying, he still had absolutely no luck. I had to leave the room. I could not bear to listen to her scream for another minute. I could not tolerate seeing another needle go through a vein. I could not stand seeing an additional tourniquet on another sight and yet another try. I thought I was going to go mad, start to scream and never stop. No one wanted to have to get a surgeon to make an incision into either the anticubital notch on the inside of her elbow or her leg to put in a cutdown, least of all, John Tkach. Two hours after he started, he came out and announced he had finally hit a small scalp vein, and it was done. He was soaked to the skin and red faced, but he had succeeded. He left at eleven that night.

Later that night, as I was wandering the halls, trying to catch a breeze, I walked back from the cafeteria and found him in Heather's room. She was awake and playing with him. He was making funny faces and funny noises and she was laughing and having a ball. I watched them silently, not wanting to disturb them. He played with her for about twenty minutes, then sat quietly in the darkened room, and waited for her to go back to sleep. He straightened his tie, put on his suit coat, came out of the room and went home. I don't think he ever knew that I saw the two of them, and if he did, I feel certain he would deny it. He seemed, to me, to always want to appear the consummate professional and somewhat detached from emotions. I think the detached and professional guise is the only face he showed to many of his patients and their parents, but I knew better.

Chapter Nineteen

There was one breakthrough we thought was going to solve all of our problems. It was the first real sign of hope, and we all jumped on board as though it was the last lifeboat from the Titanic. One of the most eminent of the researchers working to find a treatment was Dr. Alfred Smith, in New York City. Dr. Smith had been one of he foremost authorities on Dysautonomia, and one of the research projects he was working on was drug therapy, and this promised to be the answer to our prayers. He had been experimenting with the side effects of the drug, urecholine. This had principally been used in the treatment of Myasthenia Gravis, a disease that causes a progressive loss of muscle use. He had discovered that Myasthenics were having side effects that seemed to be exactly what dysautonomics needed. He noted there was an increase in eye moisture and a better ability to generate some reflex responses. The drug worked on supplementing the acetylcholine that was so lacking in the Dysautonomic. Acetylcholine is a neurotransmitter that enables nerve impulses to bridge the neural synapse. Once we heard this, we were literally in the car and drove to New York.

In Dr. Axelrod's office it was decided Heather's eye problems were sufficiently serious to warrant a trial of the drug. The FDA did not approve it and we had to sign sheaves of waivers and consent forms to legally allow her to be one of the experimental subjects. When we got home we started the treatment immediately. Urecholine had to be injected four times a day subcutaneously. I had never used a needle before and was very apprehensive about actually sticking a needle into my child four times a day.

We had arranged for a RN from Visiting Nurses to come up and teach me how to prepare the syringes and actually inject them. Learning to draw up the medication was the easiest part. Learning to identify the proper injection sites was a snap. Learning how to inject the orange was great. Then came the moment of truth, actually sticking that thing into human flesh. Bruce wanted no part of this, but he had to learn as well as I did. I figured the best way to learn was to inject myself with sterile water, so I would become familiar with the way the syringe felt and handled. I swabbed my thigh with alcohol and sat and looked at my skin for a very long time. I'd put the needle right up to it and pull it back, over and over, I'd go through this exercise, waiting for a sign that it was the right time for this torture to commence. Finally I couldn't put it off any longer. Bruce was watching, Heather was watching, Alyssa was genuinely amazed. I stabbed that thing into my thigh, pulled back on the plunger as I had been taught, and finally injected myself with one full cc of sterile water. My immediate reaction was amazement. Sticking the needle in didn't hurt, but that damned sterile water stung like hell.

Bruce's response to this was to take a needle, fill it, and go right for my thigh. This man was no fool, if he could find someone stupid enough to let him try this, he was going to go for it. Lucky him, that stupid person was right in front of him. It is an ever-trusting woman who allows her husband to go at her with a needle. I love him dearly, but his touch with a syringe left a lot to be desired. I think he was enjoying it a little too much.

Eventually, needlework became second nature. We would inject her four times a day and hope for the best. She put up with our incompetence for as long as she could, then announced emphatically "NO MORE NEETLES." I called Dr. Smith. It was then that he told me the medication was also available in pill form. Had he been there, he might have been a homicide victim. Happily, we switched from the injected medication to the pill form. Swallowing pills was impossible for Heather, so we had to pulverize the pills and mix it into her food.

The bad news was the urecholine never worked for her. The only visible effect that it had, was that it obliterated any of the bladder control she had fought so hard to attain. It had taken almost three years to toilet train her, and now at the age of four, she had to go back into diapers. We gave up on the urecholine after about six months convinced it was not the wonder cure we had prayed for. Instead it had caused another set of problems.

Chapter Twenty

When Heather was well, she spent five mornings a week at preschool. A curriculum had been devised to address her unique learning disabilities and target the educational areas that required the most intense work. Her fine motor coordination was severely compromised by her body's lack of proprioception. She lacked the ability to know what her body was doing or where it was in space. She had to be taught to pay attention to the details of what she was doing to successfully complete a project. Her hands always tended to move before she knew what she wanted them to do. We found using puzzles helped her learn to be deliberate when trying to control her manual dexterity. She learned precision by making the puzzle pieces fit only after carefully studying the shapes and then thinking before selection of the proper piece and manipulation to make it conform to the empty shape in the puzzle form. Things that happened automatically for normal children had to become learned behaviors for Heather.

She was very apprehensive when other children approached her. She was used to the smooth and precise movements of adults and trusted them, but preschool aged children's movements were often herky jerky and this made her nervous. One of the most enormous challenges she had to address in school was having to learn to be comfortable in the company of other children her own age.

When children are chronically sick, their socialization is very different from that of healthy children. They become accustomed to the rigorous routines of hospital life. Going outside to play was a perilous endeavor, not good clean fun. Play was one of the most important social challenges Heather tried to meet. Adults played with her and always made her the center of their attention. She had always been the focus, and she had to learn to be peripheral. School taught her to be patient with other children and it also taught her to be child-like. Seemingly routine play behaviors were totally alien to her. The simple act of going down a slide brought her amazing joy. It took weeks for her to learn to go down the slide and trust enough to take her hands off the edges, but it was worth the effort when she succeeded.

We measured her successes in terms of smiles. When she finally mastered an unusually hard behavior, she had a sense of accomplishment. She was proud to be able to play and not be singled out as something even more unusual than she was. Of course we always had to be constantly vigilant of injury, or that too much wind that might dry out her eyes. She could never play alone, but she could play.

In all of the literature we had read about Dysautonomia, it was not clear whether traditional education would ever work, and since so few of the children survived into adulthood, they were hard pressed to elaborate on the what worked and how it was best implemented. We were breaking new ground. With each child studied, information was acquired that would contribute to a pool of information and techniques that would attempt to make the educational process easier for children subsequently diagnosed.

Educationally, Heather's focus was on speech.

Before she could learn anything else, she had to become intelligible to the outside world. The mislocations of her tongue were always a dominant problem. She simply did not perceive it in her mouth. Once she bit her tongue so severely, it looked like a very rare steak that had been cut halfway through. Luckily, the tongue heals quickly. My heart almost jumped out of my chest when she stuck her tongue out to me and tried to say "boo-boo Mommy."

It was critical to make her aware of where her tongue was and what it was doing. In speech therapy she would sit in front of a mirror with her speech therapist, Carol Miller, and stick out her tongue and move up and down and from side to side. Carol was a student at Worcester State College and Heather loved her very much. She wanted to look like Carol and loved to dress up in "big girl clothes, like Calal." Because of her rapport with Carol Miller, Heather's speech sessions were smooth and enjoyable. Had she not enjoyed the lessons so much, she never would have been patient enough to repeat the tongue and mouth exercises hour after hour.

In the spring of 1975, Dr. Anna Cohen, director of the Worcester State College Department of Communication Disorders, and also the driving force behind the Collaborative Pre-School that Heather attended, had a brilliant idea. She wanted to work with the Audio-Video Department and create a new teaching method. She wanted them to bring into being and produce a documentary about Heather and use to as a teaching device. Videography was a relatively new art form and we had never realized that it was a much easier media form to use than old-fashioned movie cameras and editing techniques.

Anna wrote a grant and convinced the powers that be, at Worcester State College, there would never be a better opportunity to showcase the Speech and Language Department in general and Heather in particular. They would, in all likelihood, never again encounter a case like Heather's and it was, in her opinion, an amazing opportunity.

When she approached us, we were apprehensive. This would mean having a videographer, producer, and various technicians invading our home for weeks. They wanted to watch us doing all of our usual routines, and conduct interviews. They wanted to interrogate us. They wanted to confer with other parents, friends, doctors, teachers and so on. This little videotape was evolving all by itself and reinventing itself on a daily basis. It was becoming a major production that was revolving around Heather.

Heather was very photogenic and a natural ham.

She mugged for the camera and thoroughly enjoyed herself. They taped her at home, school and speech therapy. The only things they didn't tape were the three or four hospitalizations that occurred during production. Those horrors did not need the further confusion of a camera crew.

We recreated her fourth birthday for the video, complete with cake. Gathering around the dining room table, Bruce, Alyssa and I sang Happy Birthday, no less than five times. Either the lighting was off, or the audio didn't pick up, or there was a shot of the kitchen inadvertently in the scene or a technical problem. There were shoots and re-shoots of all of the scenes. Heather thought this was great, and started using the taping as an excuse for her doing anything she pleased.

If I told her to pick up her toys, she would put her hands on her hips and announce, "Me no do dat. Me movie star." After a while that started to wear very thin on all of us. One afternoon as she was announcing her status as the next Elizabeth Taylor, I got fed up with her and told her that she was not, in fact, a movie star, she was a little shit, and not to forget it.

A couple of days later, when the camera crew was taping an interview in our living room, Heather strolled into the room and happily announced, "Me no movie star. Me liddle chit." She was just as happy to be a "liddle chit" as she was to be a movie star, as long as she was the only one and she could get a laugh from it.

Alyssa in the meantime was having as much fun with this little project as Heather was. She was an unconstrained producer and director. She dragged the cameraman all over the house, showing him her guinea pig, appropriately named the Filthy Beast, or played the electric organ. She tried her level best to take over as producer of the film. Her biggest problems were what would she wear for a particular shot, and how should she wear her hair. One ponytail, pigtails or down straight. She selected Heather's outfits as well. We never could do anything without her. She took over and directed anyone who would let her.

The amazing thing about this project was its result. Yes, it was very effective as a teaching tool. It gave a very intimate look at a family trying the best it could just to keep body and soul together. But it was more than that. It generated a tremendous amount of community interest and involvement. The newspapers resurrected their old stories about his unusual child, and what happened next was that the community got on board and everyone wanted to see this modest little project that had evolved into an event.

On the night, in January 1976 that "WITHOUT TEARS" had been scheduled to premiere at Worcester State College, hundreds of people showed up to see it. No one expected that kind of response. As the auditorium filled, it became clear there were many more people than seats. The audio-visual staff scrambled to tie in all of their video equipment. Monitors were set up in lecture halls and classrooms and, at that, not all were accommodated. Standing in the lobby of the building that housed the auditorium, Bruce and I were flabbergasted by the volume of traffic that wanted to see a story about our daughter. We wondered if it was mere curiosity, or more than that?

When the film was over, men and women had tears in their eyes and there was thunderous applause. Both Alyssa and Heather were there and it was as though they had both made their Broadway debuts. Heather was radiant in her triumph. Alyssa exhibited her star quality of magnanimous modesty that has served her so well through the years. Bruce and I were happy that it was over and we could try to get back to life as usual.

Chapter Twenty One

The summer 1976 was a slow motion nightmare. Heather was having horrid bouts of aspiration pneumonia and she was not responding to any of the usual medications and antibiotics. Her veins were so badly scarred that getting IVs into her was becoming a practical impossibility. No sooner had someone hit a vein than it would collapse. They tried her arms, hands, feet, ankles, scalp and nothing would support a line.

As her fevers grew higher and higher, cut-downs had to be employed. As the first cut-down was made, the surgeon was busy with the local anesthetic and finding the precise location to cut into her arm and insert the intravenous catheter. I tried to comfort her as best I could, but she was sick and tired of people touching her and bothering her. I had to keep her still while the procedure was being done. Seeing a surgeon slice into the inside of her arm made me feel both weak and nauseated, but there was no choice. I had to stay there to comfort her, and somehow, I had to manage to stay on my feet and not pass out cold. I had seen hundreds of IVs started and the sight of the blood had never bothered me, but the sight of him severing her flesh and digging deep enough to get a good vein, was almost too much to take. Drenched with perspiration, light-headed and dead pale, I had to stand and watch as still one more "thing" was being done to my child

We had to pack her armpits and groin with ice. As she lay on the cooling blankets shivering and screaming to make it stop, we knew we could not. They had placed a rectal temperature probe, and it measured the numbers that seemed impossible to survive. Her temp was hovering between 106 and 107.6. No one knew how much more of this she could take before there was brain damage. We'd alternate doses of Tylenol and aspirin every two hours and did the best that we could to keep her hydrated. Just as quickly as it would zoom up, it would start to drop. Within twenty minutes of a fever of 106, her body temperature would fall to 95. No one had ever seen anything that had even remotely resembled what was happening. We'd pull off the ice and cover her with heated blankets and try to get her temp up. This up and down elevator ride went on for days. She would seem to be a little better then up the fever would spike again.

She could never be left alone for a minute because the fluctuations of her vital signs were so wild. That entire summer was like a bad dream. There seemed to be no way to stabilize her, and the spirals were ravaging her body. No matter how bizarre, any suggestion or idea was tried. Clearly this had to stop before it killed her.

Well into the middle of the summer, Heather was not only blowing IV lines, but cut-downs as well. The scars on her arms had started to look like roadmaps. As I recall, she would become marginally well enough to leave the hospital for a few days or a week, then relapse and have to be readmitted with still another aspiration pneumonia. Week after week, this went on, from June to September.

All of us were totally exhausted, physically, mentally, and emotionally. We were getting on one another's frayed nerves and the tension ran through the house like a tiny field mouse, insidiously moving from room to room in the stillness of night. Our collective patience was running out. We snapped at each other and silently railed at ourselves in guilt for feeling human. There were endless days and nights that simply ran into one another. By the end of September, Heather had come home. But she was very tired and weak. Her appetite returned to her slowly. I can't remember when mine came back. One more time we had cheated our ways back from death, and felt that no matter how bad things got, they couldn't possibly be any worse than they had been that summer.

For my part, I was sure I had the power to will my daughter to live, and all I had to do was to work hard enough and any problem could be managed, or at the very least survived. I had, after all, laid arrogant hands on Heather and pulled her back from death more times than I wanted to think about.

During the spring of 1976 we decided we were outgrowing our house. As Heather was amassing more and more medical equipment, we were running out of space. We had found a piece of land on the other side of Paxton that we all loved. It was a corner lot, with many varieties of trees on a very quiet street. It was the most beautiful piece of land we had seen and we instantly fell in love with it. We had to borrow $10,000. from my Uncle Si, to pay for it, but it was ours. All during the summer, the arborists cleared the trees from the land and the builder was beginning to come up with plans that fit our requirements. We had purchased the blue prints from one of the New York papers, and only had to make a few adjustments for the house to perfectly accommodate our special needs.

The exterior of the house was English Tudor, complete with gingerbread trim. The floor plans were contemporary, roomy and spacious. There were four bedrooms upstairs with one full and one half bath. The plan for downstairs called for a living room, dining room, kitchen, powder room and small family room. Outside there was a large covered patio area. The changes that we had made included dropping the living room down one step, for a sunken living room, and moving the fireplace from the living room to the family room. The family room, we enlarged by expanding its space into what had originally been the covered patio area. This allowed us to also expand the kitchen into what originally had been the family room area, effectively doubling the space both in the kitchen and the family room The floor plan for the kitchen was then adjusted to give it more work space and an open traffic flow. Through the kitchen sliding door was a small open deck area. Carved in between the kitchen and the garage, we stuck a small utility area for the washer and the dryer to get them out of the basement. The family room that we added had a high cathedral ceiling and we dropped this room down one step to make it a sunken room also. Construction began in November when they poured the foundation and the footings.

Our first house had been on the market since the summer, but no one had been interested. As the fall wore on we were allowing ourselves to relax a little about Heather as we were becoming more concerned about selling the old house.

By late November, Heather was back in school a few days a week. Sharon, my best friend and Heather's nurse found out that she was pregnant with her fourth child. This baby we joked about, wondering if it was going to hand her IUD to the obstetrician upon delivery. But, all in all, Sharon, Ron and the girls were happy, as we were for them. Alyssa looked forward to actually seeing a normal baby and mothering it as much as the Luftig girls did. I felt both sad and envious. Our decision about more children had all ready been made when Heather was an infant and we had been faced with the appalling genetic statistics. There would be no happy mistakes in our house. Once again, I mourned for the future children who were not to be.

Sharon, who had become diabetic during her pregnancy, and had back problems, did not have an easy time in her pregnancy and was unable to continue as Heather's nurse/escort. She had always been invaluable, as a friend both in need and in deed. Without Sharon as Alyssa's stand in mother, Heather's nurse and my friend, life would have been unendurable.

We interviewed dozens of RNs that were acceptable to the Special Education Department, and some that were tolerable to Heather and were finally able to hire a new nurse who was satisfactory to all of us. Her name was Margaret. She was very different from Sharon and I don't know if

Heather ever really adjusted to her. Margaret was more professional acting and less Mommy-like than Sharon was.

Chapter Twenty Two

In December of 1976 Heather was back in St. V's. This time she was vomiting blood. The only explanation for this was she had to be bleeding into her stomach. I had never seen anything like this before, and it was terrifying. They had passed a naso-gastric tube into her stomach to pump out the blood and hydrochloric acid. She was feverish and hysterical and not comprehending any of what was going on around her. They were suctioning out liter after liter of blood and acid. No one could understand how she was producing so much stomach acid, but it was making it impossible for her stomach lining to heal. What this disease did not diminish, it exaggerated. There seemed to be no end to the new and different dirty little tricks Heather's body was playing on itself.

The only explanation we could come up with for the bleeding was that she had now developed stress ulcers. Nothing else made sense. As before, her veins would not support any of the intravenous needles, so still another cut down had to be done. The only comfort she could have was one of us holding her hands and reading to her while they were making the incisions in her arm and trying to thread in the catheter. We could not pick her up much for fear of blowing the cut down. When she slept we ate or slept.

Although she had bleeding stress ulcers in her stomach, she felt no pain and still wanted to eat. Whenever she saw or smelled food for another patient, she would scream and carry on, demanding her meals. I would look her straight in the eye and lie to her about being able to eat soon, knowing at best we were talking about days or weeks, not minutes or hours.

As we were about to begin construction on the house, there were decisions that had to be made. Most of these decisions were made in the conference room on the 7th floor of St. V.'s. Frequently in the afternoons, our builder, a sensitive and gentle man, named Ed Piel would drive downtown, blueprints in hand, and try to discuss construction options. I remember planning the layout of the kitchen in that conference room. The amazing thing is that we did not make any major mistakes. In retrospect, there was only one recognizable flaw. There are six doors including the ones to the garage, basement, broom closet, two bi-folds that cover the laundry area and the one that leads into the entry hall, that all open inward. When one door is open, it is impossible to open any of the others without closing the first one. Small details.

Heather's stomach did not want to heal. Days dragged on, and she was still bleeding into her belly. She could not eat and her disposition was becoming sour and agitated. She wanted to know why everyone else could eat and she could not. She could smell the food from the dietary carts and shriek in fury and disappointment.

As healing finally began slowly, the amount of stomach acid started to ebb. As mid December grew closer to Christmas, she gradually started to feel better. By the third week of December, she was able to drink milkshakes and eat Jell-O. Every day I would promise her cheesecake the following day, and Mac Donald's soon after that. We promised her anything. Apple pie was to be on the menu the day before she was discharged. With as much patience as a five-year old could muster, she waited it out.

The day before she was discharged, we brought up a huge apple pie, and all of the pediatric intensive care staff shared it with Heather. We had battled and won still another war.

Chapter Twenty Three

There were snow flurries in the morning on February 2, 1977. A major snowfall had not been predicted, yet I felt increasingly more apprehensive about driving. Blizzards had never bothered me, I could drive through just about anything, but there was something very different going on, that day. I was feeling extremely fearful and jumpy, so I called the Paxton Police Department and asked them to give Heather and me a ride down to St. V.'s. Heather was not sick, but she had a low-grade temp of 99 degrees. She had no symptoms, and was acting like her usual playful self. Still, I felt a disquieting and remarkable unease.

Driving downtown in the police cruiser, Heather had a grand time playing with the buttons, siren and radio in the police car. She was so charming and delightful, in fact, the officer let her sit on his knee at stop-lights. She was having a perfectly wonderful time. I was chewing on my nails and chain smoking through the slightly opened window.

When I brought her up to the seventh floor pediatric unit, the director in charge could not understand why we were there. He examined her and then flatly told me to take her home and deal with what ever it was by myself. I explained to him that I did not have a car and it would be a real problem, not to mention the fact I was sure she was coming down with something and I wanted her where she was.

After a twenty minute argument, he agreed to let her stay overnight, and then I would have to take her home in the morning when nothing developed. I nodded my assent.

While she was eating her supper, she was in a very nasty and uncooperative state, and I really did not want to have a lot to do with her when she was acting like such a brat and being so troublesome. When I told her that I would read her one story and then it would be bedtime, she complained. I read her still another story. She went to sleep.

I kissed her forehead and she felt cool to my touch.

I had some more coffee and a few more cigarettes and schmoozed in the unit office until about 11:30, then found an empty bed down at the end of the hall, and went to sleep myself.

The charge nurse shook me awake at 2:30 am. I looked at her in amazement. This was something she had never done before. Heather, she said as gently as possible, had had a grand mal seizure about twenty minutes before, and they could not stop it. I raced to her room panic stricken.

Heather was shaking uncontrollably on the bed. They had given her Phenobarbital, Dilatin and Thorazine. Nothing was working. Her breathing was erratic. They wanted to intubate her and put her on a ventilator. They wanted to do a lumbar puncture. They wanted more blood cultures. Yes, yes, yes do it all, was all that I could manage to say. Bruce had been called and he was on his way, after dropping Alyssa at the Luftig's doorstep.

When the seizure stopped, Heather was in a coma. Neurologists dug their thumbs into her breastbone looking for a deep pain response, not realizing even in her normal state would there be none, got no response. Nothing happened. No matter what anyone did, nothing happened. She just lay there motionless. We read to her, we talked to her, we screamed at her to wake up, but there was nothing.

By daybreak, we were all in shock trying to figure out what had just happened. But there were no answers. Carl and Sylvia called my mother and Bruce's sister. My mother called my brother and my aunts and uncles.

They were all driving or flying in that day. We had no answers, only questions. The CT scan showed cerebral edema, indicating that her brain was swelling. They started running diuretics through her cut down trying in desperation to reduce the fluid pressure in her head.

By the end of the day, they were having problems with the ventilator and wanted to do a tracheotomy and ventilate her through that. We asked a friend who was an ENT if he would perform the surgery for the trach, and he agreed and took her to surgery that night. An hour after they took her down to the surgical suite, her trach was in place, and there was no change in her condition.

Days were running into one another, her status remained the same. She was critical, comatose and unresponsive.

Her EEG was not promising.

John Tkach came in every morning and every night. It did not matter what we tried. He called in Neuro consults from the U Mass Medical Center, and they too were at a loss. We conference called NYU, daily, but none of their suggestions worked. Once the cerebral edema had subsided, she should have regained consciousness. But she didn't. Then her lungs started to fail.

At some point during that week, I was trying to get some sleep on the sofa in the 7th floor lounge, when my brother came over and sat next to me. He felt it was his duty and obligation to try to prepare me. I knew his intent was to give me some support and ease the tension, but I did not want to hear his words. I did not want to be forced to acknowledge the obvious. I did not want to think about it.

How could he possibly appreciate the depth of the grief and anguish that I was feeling? There was nothing in his frame of reference with which to equate it. He had no right to prepare me. This was something I had to do for myself, inevitably. I was the one who had to come to terms with it.

Whenever we walked into Heather's room in the intensive care unit, our hearts were palpitating and our throats were dry and sore from the tightness of the restraint that we had to show. Horrendous pressures moved in the hallway outside the unit. Other parents seemed to sense our pain, and walked a little quieter and held their children a little closer when they had to traverse that fifty-foot stretch of corridor.

Bruce was at the hospital day and night. Some friends came up to see us, but there was little we wanted to say to them, and even less we wanted to hear. There was no comfort for either of us. The pain and sorrow mounted by the minute. We'd sit, hour after hour, hoping, praying, making deals with an unresponsive god. We talked to Heather, sang to Heather, and begged her to open her eyes to us. We looked somberly at anyone who approached us.

One doctor, a member of the surgical house staff, came to us on the fifth day. I had never met him before and hadn't a clue who he was. Along with him was the new rotation of surgical interns and residents, like his own personal entourage and cheering squad. Our daughter's cutdown was blown and, in essence, her arm was dying.

"The tissue in her arm is becoming necrotic and developing gangrene. If she lives," he noted coldly, "we'll have to amputate her arm."

I screamed at him: "GET OUT GET OUT GET OUT." How dare he put our bare, ragged edges on display like some kind of insensitive lesson to be taught? Just go away and leave us alone. We'd do what we had to do, if and when we had to do it.

I felt a bitter loathing for that surgeon and hoped he never had the callous disregard for the parents of another dying child he had displayed with us. To him, it was another case. To us, it was our child, a child we had battled heaven and earth to keep together, care for and love. Didn't he know what he was doing to us? Or didn't he care? I hated that man, whoever he was.

In the end, early in the morning of February 10,1977 Heather's body simply gave out when her lungs could no longer oxygenate her blood sufficiently to sustain her life. I held her when she died. I smoothed her hair, and kissed her hands and face. I don't think I cried. There were no tears left. I do not remember how I got home. But I do remember waking my mother and telling her, then waking Alyssa and telling her that her sister was gone. I lied and told her something comforting about angels in heaven, not believing a single word of it. And after that, I simply shut down.

I don't remember much about the days that followed. I no longer cared. In 1976 I had written a poem about Heather.

> Her face is electric
> Impulses radiate
> Smiling, I see her all of the time.
> Her face is a spark of sun.
> She shines her love
> It comes in waves upon me
> As on a beach.
>
> Her face is light from the sun.
> How could anything so perfect be so imperfect?
> She is beauty, truth, innocence.
> She is mine always, in all ways.
> She brings me joy and pain.
> Her face is light, electric and glowing.
> And I love her so.

The first four lines of this poem are carved into her marker, along with the words: Heather Beth Swirsky,
February 10, 1977. Age 5 and a half.

Chapter Twenty Four

As bad as I thought things had been during the months that had preceded Heather's death, they never approached the horrible, gaping, sucking vacuum, which ensued after she died. When you go from a situation that totally controls every waking moment of your life into one that requires no conscious thought at all, uselessness and malaise fill in the voids. Transitioning your entire system into another is a pain-filled and debilitating task. I knew what I was capable of and suddenly those capacities were on hold, empty and stuck in a lethargic blankness, no future and an unthinkable past. If life for the past five years could have been defined as total envelopment, this was it's polar opposite. How was I supposed to deal with it? If I had known the answer, if only I had known that one.

The days that followed the funeral found me in a complete shutdown. When someone said sit, I sat. If they said get dressed, I got dressed. When they said it was time to eat, I'd shove the food around on my plate and look at it. The sight of food on a plate was both repulsive and nauseating. That I had another child did not matter. That I had a husband who was hurting every bit as much as I did, did not matter. That I had a house in construction and another one that had to be sold didn't matter. I no longer cared. That I lived another day did not matter. My purpose was gone. There was nothing that could fill my hours and give me a reason to exist. The pain was total and unforgiving. Being conscious of it was unrelenting, excruciating and debilitating.

I would go to the cemetery and sit in the snow and weep. When I left the cemetery, soaked to the skin and shivering, I would go on autopilot and try to drive home. Being near her was the only small, cold comfort I could allow myself. Never, had I dreamed so much pain was possible. Surely this had to be beyond human endurance.

In attempts at comfort, friends came to the house and tried to visit. I would sit and stare past them. It was too much effort to converse. There was nothing they could say to me that I wanted to hear. There was, on my part, no response possible, only an exanimate and empty expression around my eyes. I knew, intellectually that Alyssa was in pain, but there was no consolation in me to give to her. She was left to deal with her pain, as best any seven-year old could. She did not understand her sister was dead, and her mother was as good as dead.

She reversed roles and tried to comfort and shelter me. She would bring me the mail, tell me to eat, or bathe, she told me when she thought I should take a nap. She brought home no friends, and played little. February and March were slow motion nightmares playing themselves out for our collective benefits.

One cold and particularly lousy Saturday in April, Sharon, Ron, Miriam, Aimee and Gillian Luftig came to the house and dragged Alyssa and me to the annual Flower Show in Boston. Lys had a wonderful time running in and out of the flowers and displays with Gillian. I barely noticed the colors all around me. When they dropped us off, late in the afternoon, Lys was happy and flushed with excitement about the wonderful day she had had. I do remember that I was able to force myself to enthuse about the show, but not much.

Bruce wrapped himself up in his work and dealt with his loss by himself, together, we were unable to console one another.

As April played out, the house finally sold. I had to force myself to pack our belongings in preparation for our move across town into the new house. I soon became obsessed with getting out of the old house and into the new one. Being in the old house was intolerable.

Although construction was not yet complete, there was heat, electric and water and I had to move. It was as if the old house and its ghosts refused to allow me to breathe. The day we moved, April 15, 1977, it sleeted and snowed intermittently. It did not matter. There were workmen all over the place, alternately fighting with the movers and helping them, so that they would be finished sooner and get out of the way. We moved into bare, freshly plastered walls, no carpets, and no bathtub or shower fixtures. There was sub flooring throughout the house except where the tile had been laid in the kitchen and bathrooms. There was no driveway, only mud, no banisters on the stairs, and no cupboards in the kitchen, but I was relieved to be out of the old house and away from its memories. I physically was not able to walk into the room that was to have been Heather's, and that door stayed closed.

There was dust and mud all over everything. The place was a mess and that, at least, gave me a short-term purpose. I cleaned. I vacuumed. I swept. There were opportunities to forget, at least for a few minutes at a time. But when the work was done, the memories flooded back. I relived the last week of Heather's life every time I closed my eyes. I'd see her face looking at me with hope and trust, the way she had looked at me when we said good night to one another the last time, before the seizure.

One afternoon, I had to drive north across Route 31 into the town of Holden. That stretch of road traverses the Kendall Reservoir. As I silently approached the water, I had the conscious thought that if I drove into the reservoir on the right side, it would look intentional, but if I drove off on the left side, it would look a though I had lost control of the car. The water looked very inviting, under all of the newly melting ice. It was silent, cold and an excellent exit. They could never pull me out in time. I remember all of these thoughts as though it was yesterday. I also remember the very conscious thought of what that would do to Bruce and Alyssa.

Did I really have the right to do that to them? I stopped the car on the side of the road. As I sat there shaking, I realized for the first time how truly despondent I was and that I needed help to try to salvage the rest of my life. More to the point, I had to choose if I wanted to live.

Out of the necessity to save my life, I found help. Three times a week, for six weeks and I began to give myself permission to feel again. At least for a little at a time. There was a true despair at work and it had done its damage. This depression was not one borne of chemical or psychosocial roots. It was the one left in the wake of profound, visceral sadness and loss.

It took less time than I had imagined to sort out the grief. Perhaps this was because there truly was no guilt to be felt. In every way possible, I fought for Heather's life. I was, I learned, a lousy loser. I had to learn I was not omnipotent and there were some things I simply could not fix. Having been forced into a role of a domineering power freak to save my child, it was not a station I wanted to ever consider relinquishing. I had pulled her back from death so many times that it had never occurred to me that at some time I would not be able to do it any longer, and this was not anything over which I had control. I had not only lost my child; I had lost my power. Power had become my drug of choice: my crutch.

Chapter Twenty Five

As summer came, I worked my way out of a tunnel, and into the dim light at the end. There were moments that were sheer nightmares. The first time I saw a dark haired, dark eyed little girl of about Heather's age and size, I literally ran screaming from the waiting room of my dentist's office. I could not look at her.

I'd wake up from real nightmares in which Heather would beg me to take her home. I also dreamed of being buried alive. In time they were less frequent.

On the day of Heather's unveiling, the ritual of uncovering the monument at the cemetery, and the official end of the mourning period in the Jewish religion, I found myself unable to swallow. Every piece of solid food I put into my mouth felt like it was cemented to the wall of my throat. I thought there was a logjam in my esophagus. Nothing went past it. I called my therapist. He told me that I had that I had that particular symptom because it had specifically been one of Heather's worst problems and subconsciously I was trying to duplicate the situations I had lived through.

I thought that was a crock of shit, and told him so. He told me I was entitled to my opinion. I took some Valium to get through the day, and somehow managed to make it.

Chapter Twenty Six

In September of 1977, I got a call from one of Alyssa's dancing teachers. Another girl Alyssa had danced with had died of Cystic Fibrosis. Would I come and talk to the mother? How could I do that? How could I tell Alyssa? Could she bear another explanation beyond her comprehension? Driving down the hill from Paxton into Worcester to see the family was numbing. There was nothing I could say to this woman to ease her pain. There was less I could do to give her comfort. I was barely holding on myself. I remember walking up the stairs in to the house feeling like my legs were stuck in concrete, and questioning how anyone could be crazy enough to think I could possibly give comfort. What I could not understand was that she took comfort in the fact that I had survived. The best I could do was to be there and to cry together.

What surprised me the most was Alyssa. She took in the news about Elisa's death and had very little reaction. At the time, I did not understand what was happening. Later, I did, all too well. She had asked me about what had happened, and I explained that Elisa had a very rare disease, much like Heather, and much like Heather it was too hard for her body to fight any longer. It was, I said, a one in a million thing and nothing like that was ever going to happen to her. Things like this were very, very, very rare and she did not have to worry, because only very sick children ever died. She accepted this and cried little. She got on about her life, as resilient as ever.

A month or so after Elisa died, Alyssa slipped and fell on the stairs in our new house and hooked her foot in the banister. Although there was no swelling or bruising, she was making such a fuss I had to take her to the Emergency Room of our local hospital. The pain was terrible, she said, and she could not walk on it. The doctor there examined her foot and ankle and sent her for x-rays. They were negative. The on-call resident said there was absolutely nothing worse than a slight twist and bruise and to give her Tylenol and send her to school. After all, he was the doctor, and he knew what he was talking about.

She complained constantly about her foot and how much it hurt her, and I explained that sprains were often painful and that there really wasn't much that could be done about it except take the Tylenol, tape it up and get on with it.

Still she complained continually. That was not like her at all. I found myself second-guessing. Was this an attention getting device? The thought occurred to me that maybe she was pulling a number on me. Certainly that was imaginable. She hadn't mourned for her sister, or Elisa, maybe this was the display of unexpressed emotion.

I was vacillating between my opinions. Should I take her to a counselor instead of back to the doctor? After all, the doctor had said that she was fine.

Two or three days after the fall, I got a call from the school nurse. Did I know that my daughter was hopping from class to class and going up the stairs on her knees? I certainly had no idea.

After agonizing all afternoon and wondering if she was really hurt or if it was a ploy for some attention, I called orthopedics at Umass Med Center and asked to speak to Dr. Arthur Pappas, the orthopedist that had treated Heather. He said to pick up her x-rays and bring her right down. He took one look at the x-rays, then put his hand on her ankle to examine it. She screamed in agony. She had laterally separated the ligament in her right ankle and was in a cast using crutches for eight weeks.

That accident, the self-doubt and fear on my part was a wake up call. Get off your ass and start to listen to yourself, not anyone else. Believe your gut. I had, temporarily, lost the ability to trust my own instincts. I had begun to doubt my every word and action. The immobilization that had begun on the night Heather had died, had totally undermined my entire sense of being, warped my mind and consequently maimed every aspect of my personality.

Chapter Twenty Seven

It became my mission to try to survive. In my survival, I had to reestablish the link to Alyssa I had lost. I had to save not only myself, but her as well. In recognition of this came still another danger. Could I allow myself to suck her up to fill my void? Once more came the battles. In my heart I wanted to protect her and shelter her from all of the pain and danger in life. In my mind I could only recognize fear and the peril inherent in trying to do this. She had survived her sister's death. Now it was time for her to survive her mother.

I went into armed combat with my emotions every time she wanted to go out on her bicycle or walk to a friend's house that was more than 100 feet down the street. I no longer believed that my child was safe. I feared every danger, real and imagined. I wanted to be there and protect her from life. The first time she fell off her bike, I panicked. Every time she caught a cold and ran a fever, I had visions of febrile convulsions. She started to have a problem with an allergic cough. I was not to be satisfied until she was worked up for everything from hay fever to pleurisy to asthma. I considered asking John Tkach to look for lung cancer, but finally regained control over my panic. My over-reactions were epic in scope. While I battled my fears and demons, I had to try to bite my tongue and say nothing, or as little as possible.

During this period, Bruce once made the mistake of mentioning he thought possibly, at some point in the future, we might adopt another child. I went ballistic. How could he think I would dream of replacing my dead child? I would not hear of it. Heather had been dead less than eight months, and he had the nerve to consider adoption. That was, I thought, one of the most heartless and inhuman things I had ever heard.

Chapter Twenty Eight

Christmas season that year was hellish. Although we were Jewish, Bruce's women's clothing business dictated that we deal with Christmas. As in the past, Bruce had to work every night until nine o'clock, and Sundays from Thanksgiving to Christmas Eve. If this entire year had been complete wretchedness, this was the cherry on top. There was nowhere to go to escape Christmas. Alyssa was trying hard to be merry and to enjoy the first Christmas season that she could remember having her mother around. I was trying hard to survive from one hour to the next. Whenever there were Christmas carols on the radio in the car, I'd remember all of those horrific, graphic Christmases in the Pedi ICU.

I remembered the year that Beth decorated Heather like a Christmas tree. I remembered the past year with it's own unique and particular horrors. The memories were all flooding through my brain nonstop, in perfect playback. I would try to focus on shopping, anything to keep me from climbing into my head and reliving the past until there was no present. I would do almost anything to stay busy and as focused as possible. It was a gargantuan, impossible task.

All the family, Carl, Sylvia, my mother, Bruce and I overcompensated and showered Alyssa with presents. Everywhere you turned Barbie Dolls and accessories, clothes, games, books and dancing things covered the floors. The area under the dining room table was then designated as Barbie-land: no adults allowed. Ballet skirts, leotards, shoes, tights, leg warmers and everything ever created for small dancers, many in duplicate and triplicate were strewn over the chairs and the floor. Our big surprise present was a trip to Florida during February vacation. Alyssa was delighted. She started to pack Christmas morning.

We survived Christmas Eve by filling our home with people. I invited everyone I could think of to come to the house. I did not want to think about the three of us sitting around alone with empty memories on Christmas Eve. We had Chinese food and stayed occupied with other people. We looked forward to the new-year. It would no longer be 1977. Thank God. This new-year of 1978, had to be a better year. It could not conceivably be worse.

Throughout all of January and the first two weeks of February the only thing Alyssa talked about was the Florida trip. She had recently informed us she had a boyfriend. In the third grade it was critical, she assured us, to be linked romantically with the cutest boy in the class. This boy, she announced, was David, her new boyfriend. When she wasn't shopping or packing her favorite Barbie dolls, she was agonizing over what she was going to buy for her new beau. When school pictures were delivered in January, she pointed to a cute little boy with brownish blonde hair and dimples. It was David this and David that and do I think that David would like this instead of that. It was endless and life affirming.

As January melted into February, I dragged myself through the worst of a harrowing month. February 10, the first anniversary of Heather's death was indescribable in its total devastation. Another monstrous twenty-four hours to try to survive. Most of the day, I sat in the dark with the lights off, and the shades down and sobbed. Although the cemetery looked like a good place to spend the day, it was about 23 degrees out with a wind chill factor of 20 below, and snowing very heavily. Instead, I sat at home in the dark and suffered in solitude.

An amazing and surprising thing was that on the eleventh, I found I could actually cope and function without too much desolation. This also was the week of the blizzard of 1978 when the entire East Coast was buried under a three-day snowfall that had begun on the tenth. The town of Paxton, in particular, was buried under the five feet of snow that fell in less than forty-eight hours. Maybe things were easier because all the neighbors on the our street were home from work and we got together and spent our time helping each other dig out and putting together enormous pot luck dinners at one another's houses. Time was finally beginning to start the healing process. Slowly, we dug out and then we had to start packing to get ready to go on vacation in the middle of the month.

Chapter Twenty Nine

The warmth of the Florida sunshine was healing and wonderful. We stayed at Carl and Sylvia's condo in Hallandale. Most of the days I sat at the pool and watched Alyssa swim and worked on a great tan. Almost all of our shopping trips revolved around Alyssa's search for the precise gift for David. This was Alyssa's Holy Grail. We went to every souvenir and junk store in south Florida. We settled for a small wooden crate of candy oranges. She was delighted with her purchase. We were happy that at least she had found something that suited her needs and met with her standards of perfection.

The trip was the tonic that we all needed to make it through another long New England winter. It only lasted ten days and we were back on the plane flying into Boston. Carl and Sylvia picked us up and we were all brown and happy. When we got home at about 9:30 that evening, the phone was ringing. It was Sharon Luftig. She wanted to get to me before Alyssa had the chance to talk to any of her friends. There was yet another tragedy with which to deal. One of the kids in the third grade class had died suddenly of Reyes Syndrome. He had taken ill a couple of days after the flu and been taken to St. Vincent's Hospital. He had been comatose. His parents, forced to acknowledge that he was brain dead, terminated life support and donated his organs for transplantation.

"Who was this child," I asked.

Her answer sent my sprawling. It was Alyssa's new boyfriend, David. How much more could any of us take? I felt like I had been sucker punched. I told Bruce after Alyssa had gone to bed. There was no way that I could tell her that still another child that she was close to had died. I didn't know how I could expect my child to deal with this. She had been through too much already. There were no answers for the questions that I knew that she was going to ask. Tragedy simply exists. There are no reasons or explanations.

The following morning when Alyssa woke up, I told her that I had to tell her some bad news. I could not tell her yet that David had died the day before. I told her instead David had become very sick and was in the hospital. She had no reaction. She nodded and went to her room. She scared me more by this reaction that she would have if she had become hysterical. She stoically chose not to react. Later that day, I sat down with her and cautiously explained what had happened and that David had died. I told her that the odds of something like this happening were one in a million. She coolly looked at me and said,

"Just how many of these one in a million things do you think I am going to believe"

Shocked by her reaction, I had no answer. I cradled her, expecting tears and sorrow. What I got, was nothing. I did not know how I was supposed to deal with this. I was barely holding on myself and was in no condition to help her. As much as I wanted to, there was not anything I could say to comfort her. Her reaction was to withdraw and not concede to any of her feelings. She had evidently learned the way to deal with grief was to withdraw. Always the apt pupil, she had learned this lesson from her mother.

The first day of school after vacation was a nightmare. It was also the day of David's funeral. The school guidance counselor, Maryanne Morin called me.

"Did we know? How was Alyssa reacting? How were any of us coping?"

"Not well," I told her. She had called specifically to tell me that she was bringing a special grief counselor in to talk to the whole third grade class. Many of the children had also known Heather, some of the girls had also known Elisa and of course, they all had known David, as he had been one of the most popular boys in the class. None of these kids was reacting well, or normally. Alyssa's reaction was an exaggeration of the feelings and behavior that many of the other children were displaying. Although some had cried, many had also become withdrawn and were depressed.

We spoke for hours that day and she suggested that I speak to Jean Whitcomb, the wife of one of the town clergymen, who was the grief counselor that she had arranged to work with the third grade.

Jean was a gentle-hearted, comforting woman with an open and warm smile and an amazing ability to work with children in pain. She spent weeks with the whole third grade class and more weeks still with several of the children who were having the most trouble. With Alyssa, she spent the most time. We decided, during the time Jean was still working with the third graders, we would also ask her to give Alyssa private piano lessons. That was the guise, under which the counseling would take place. Jean would give Alyssa lessons, once or twice a week.

Alyssa hated playing the piano, never practiced and never got to be any good at playing, but she never complained about taking her piano lessons. At the same time, Alyssa chose to continue with her dancing lessons, her first love, and something at which she was actually getting quite good. This gave her the opportunity to physically work out some of her emotions and stress.

As spring was rushing at us, Alyssa was dancing, taking piano lessons and very busy with her activities, but not spending time with her friends. She had systematically cut her connections with her old friends. It seemed she was afraid if she got close to anyone else, she would lose him or her as well. She never had friends over to the house to play Barbie, and never went to their houses. She had been such a social child before, and since David's death, she had pulled away from all of her associations. Jean tried to explain that this was normal for a child who had been through was she had been through, but we worried just the same.

Chapter Thirty

Intermittently, Bruce mentioned adoption. It had never seemed the appropriate time to discuss it. In April of 1978, we decided this might be the right time to explore the possibilities of adoption, for many different reasons. Primary in our minds was giving Alyssa a sibling who was normal; one she could love, and laugh with, and fight with without fear that she was going to cause the baby to seize or suffer grave physical harm. She deserved a normal and healthy childhood, and so far, she had not had any semblance of one. We contacted our attorney to ask for suggestions on how best to proceed. We told him that we wanted a normal, healthy baby. No special needs, no sickness, no insurmountable problems.

He did the necessary research and suggested we consider an out of the county adoption. A domestic adoption, he told us, could take years, and we were rapidly climbing into our thirties and did not think a baby in our forties would be a very bright idea. Alyssa was eight at the time, and we did not want more than ten-year age spans in between children. We wanted an infant. International, again, was his answer. We told him to check it out and recommend how best to proceed.

By May, Alyssa was still deep in her funk. One afternoon, she came home with a kitten. She had found it and thought it was a stray. Could we keep it? We had never had cats or dogs and the thought of an animal had never occurred to us. Bruce and I told her to take it around the neighbor-hood and see if anyone claimed it. If no one did, we told her we could keep it.

She went to every house in the area, from door to door, asking if the cat belonged to anyone. None of the neighbors knew anything about this lit-tle gray and white tiger striped kitten. We thought Alyssa was home free. We should have realized the impossibility of that occurring. On the fourth day, one of our neighbors, who had been at Cape Cod for a few days, returned and claimed the kitten.

Lys was heartbroken. I begged the woman. I would buy the cat from her, pay her anything, please let my child keep the kitten. This was the first creature she had allowed herself to attach to, emotionally. As adamant as I was, the neighbor woman was more so. This cat was her teenage daughter's: a gift from her boy friend. I was furious. If she cared so much for this cat, why did she let it roam free for a week? As much as I raged on, it was to no avail.

The following afternoon after school, we canceled her "piano lesson" for the day and went to the animal shelter. Alyssa picked out a tiny, scrawny, sick looking black kitten. It was as if she intentionally selected the most pathetic looking creature in the entire shelter. In retrospect, I suppose that is exactly what she did. She never believed this kitten would live, and she was not only preparing herself for the worst, she was inviting it.

We went straight from the animal shelter to the vet. The kitten had worms, ear mites and was severely undernourished. He gave us pills for the worms, drops for the ears, vitamins and special high calorie kitten food for "Cookie", the newest member of our family. At that, he was not hopeful about Cookie's chances for survival. I gave the vet a check for $90.00 and Cookie took her chances with her new family.

When, nine years later, Cookie died of kidney failure, she died in my arms, and I cried as though I had lost my best friend. In actuality, she was more than that. She brought Alyssa back to life. She was the first warm-blooded creature that Lys allowed to enter her private empty realm.

Cookie warmed her, gave her the comfort I could not. Cookie's gift was purring, scratching, cuddly-warm sensation. She was Alyssa's lifeline. I could not understand what was happening when Alyssa got Cookie, but it was as real and palpable as any relationship I have ever seen. They were inseparable. When Alyssa went outside to play, Cookie was never more than ten feet away from her. Wherever Lys went, Cookie went. She never left our property when we let her out during the school day, and she always waited at the door when the school bus dropped Alyssa off at the end of the day. She seemed to sense Alyssa's need and gently drew her into a relationship of trust. Alyssa knew Cookie would never run away or leave her. Cookie, for her part, was true to Alyssa's expectations.

Chapter Thirty One

Life was beginning again, slowly. Our attorney called and gave us the name of agencies to contact about adoption. Once we had made up our minds to go through with the adoption, there was no stopping us. Needless to say, before we commenced our search, we consulted Alyssa and asked for her input. She was delighted. She had no idea what the adoption process was, but she thought it sounded like a good idea anyway. After all, she had just adopted a cat, how difficult could it be to adopt a baby, she reasoned.

To be on the safe side, we decided to put our names in to the local agencies as well as the international one John Keeton, our lawyer had suggested. We contacted all of the agencies in the Worcester area, and on John's advice, contacted International Adoptions in Newton, Mass. We called the Jewish Family Service: they had nothing realistic to offer us. We contacted Worcester Children's Friends Society: look at a wait of somewhere between three and ten years. In desperation, we called Catholic Charities. They said they might be able to help us if we promised to bring the child up as a practicing Catholic. That was a little difficult, we explained for a couple of marginally practicing Jews. So that was out.

We sent our application to International Adoptions in Newton and waited. They wrote back and said they thought we might be able to work together and asked to arrange an appointment for an interview.

When we drove into Newton for our initial interview, Bruce and I were so nervous we left two hours before our interview, even though Newton is less than an hour drive on the Mass Turnpike from our house, door to door. When we got there, we checked the address, located the parking area, and drove into the town of Newton to have a cup of coffee and try to relax a little. This was easier said than done. We went back to the office, parked the car and walked around the block twice. Finally it was time.

Shaking hands, with the social worker, we awkwardly introduced ourselves and immediately launched into our little song and dance about why we had decided to adopt, and why we had decided to use the international route. The two of us rambled on and on like a matched set of yammering idiots. This poor woman must have thought that we were on a twenty-four hour pass from an asylum. We talked so fast and so long, she looked dazed. She was trying frantically to keep up with her note taking, as we kept rambling on. When, at last, we had finished our tale of woe, she heaved an exhausted sigh of relief.

She said she thought that we could work together and gave us sheaves of paperwork to complete. When we had mentioned we were insisting on a healthy, Caucasian infant, she questioned our motivations. At that point, I looked her straight in the eye and told her that the last thing we wanted was another sister or brother Alyssa had to explain to anyone. We needed normalcy and wanted a baby that looked as much as possible like we did, and did not need major medical attention every day of its life. I told her also, we did not consider minor medical considerations a problem, but I could not handle another child with a horrendous life threatening disease. Minor handicaps were OK, but please, nothing major. We could not go through that again. She understood.

On her counsel, we decided the best place for us to adopt from, would be Colombia. The "market" was open for international adoptions, which translated into the fact that there were not too many political problems at the time. Colombia had thousands of abandoned and unwanted children because it was a very Catholic country and believed neither in birth control or abortion.

We proceeded to contact an attorney in Cali Colombia International Adoptions had worked with before and highly recommended. I wrote a letter to her and detailed our tale of sadness and hope and told her she had been recommended. The letters to Maria Cristina, our Colombian lawyer, were unbelievably difficult for me to write. Our caseworker carefully detailed the best style for the letter. It had to be very flowery, gushy and sweet.

We were to include pictures of the three of us, together with physical descriptions, information about our home, the neighborhood, the town and the school system. It went on and on. We were told that Maria Cristina was very good at her job, and if humanly possible, she would get us a baby that "fit" into our lives. I had never dreamed just how good she was.

When Maria Cristina's first letter arrived, I grabbed a letter opener and carefully opened the envelop to find a three page single spaced letter, all in Spanish, a language neither of us spoke. I spent hours on the phone trying to find a friend fluent in Spanish, before the bright idea occurred to me to call the local high school and beg for assistance.

Maria Cristina's letter was in the same flowery style that had been described by the caseworker. Of the three single-spaced, pages, we were able to glean one page of the useful information we needed. In essence, she said, she would help us find the "perfect" baby. She listed all of the information she needed, the documents, photographs and of course the fees and payment schedule.

We needed birth certificates, marriage certificates, finger prints, a blank Colombian Passport application, police and Interpol clearance to certify that neither of us was a felon or had any police involvement, our passport information, and of course, names in both sexes for the baby to be Christened at birth. We would have to have the child converted to

Judaism later. We had to have all of the documents stamped by the Colombian Consulate in the state in which they were issued. This meant my birth certificate and our marriage certificate had to be stamped in the New York City Consulate, as I had been born in New Jersey and that was where our wedding had been, and the New York office served New Jersey as well. Bruce's birth certificate had to be stamped in Boston. All of these papers had to be notarized and certified at the Saltenstall State Office Building in Boston. We also needed verification that we were both healthy and financially able to support another child. We had to Xerox all of our IRS returns from the previous five years.

Each page of every document had to be stamped by the appropriate consulate and state office. Every stamp had a fee, and by the time we were through, we had spent more than $500.00 in stamping fees. At one point, when Bruce was in New York City getting something or other stamped at the Colombian Consulate, the car was towed to an impound lot, as the meter had run out. Add another $150.00 to get the car back.

The hardest part of the process was picking names. Of course the baby would be named for Heather, and we decided also for Bruce's grandmother, Gussie. After weeks of indecision, and agonizing, we finally settled on Holly Gillian for a girl, and Hayden Gregory for a boy. Further, we decided if it was a boy, we would give him some time to grow into his first name of Hayden, and call him Greg.

One evening the chief of the Paxton Police Department, Dave Young, came to the house with his fingerprint kit, and printed both of us. My prints were all ready on file with the FBI, as I had worked for the State of New York as a caseworker out of the Westchester County office in Yonkers, before Alyssa had been born. It took only a few days for my prints to clear, and for some unknown reason, it took a few months for Bruce's to clear. Then, one set of prints got lost and we had to do it all over again. Between the paperwork and the busywork (like replacing the disappearing prints), we could not get all of our documents together until December of 1978. Dave Young and all of the people in the Paxton Town

Hall were wonderful. They helped get all of the documents copied, notarized, certified and properly prepared.

During this time, we went to Newton regularly for meetings with the caseworker in order for her to complete her case study. We also had to go to Newton for group meetings with other perspective parents who had also chosen to adopt from Colombia. Many times during these meetings, both Bruce and I used to wonder where it was that we sat on "THE LIST". "THE LIST" was the infamous roster of families who were working with Maria Cristina. From what we could gather, there were at least twenty families on "THE LIST." If we weren't dead last, we were damned close to it.

Many of the couples in our group were childless, and had no idea about what was involved in child raising. At one point during one of these group sessions, the caseworker asked if any of us intended to do anything actively to reinforce the child's sense of his or her heritage. Most of the younger couples launched into tirades about how they were going to do this or that to teach the child about his Spanish or Indian heritage.

Bruce, who is every bit as much of a smart mouth as I can be, said, "if you think that we are going to drape a serape over the piano and wear sombreros, you've got another thing coming. If this kid is going to be raised in a middle class Jewish family, he or she is going to be brought up as a middle class American Jewish kid, and like it. If he asks, we'll tell him what we know, and the child will always know that he's been adopted, and from where, but we cannot change what we are." That did not exactly bring cheers from our group, or group leader, but it did open up a very interesting discussion of how real life was going to enter the picture. He served as our ever-present realty check.

One afternoon in the late fall, our caseworker came to the house to make sure that we had enough room in the house for another child. They had to be sure the baby was not going to be shut away in a windowless room, and had ample space for outdoor play and activities. I had to bite my tongue and try not to tell her that our little white collar town of

Paxton was not exactly downtown Bogota, and offered every advantage anyone could ever want or dream of, and that it was outstanding in its ordinary, wonderful, down-to-earth real people. Having been born bred in Newark, New Jersey, I had a special appreciation for the differences between this town and any city. We had no smog, no noise, no buses, no air traffic, no crime, and no sirens. My worst noise complaint was that in the spring and summer when the windows were all open; a single woodpecker had the bad sense to wake me up at 5:30 am. Other than that, it was perfect. The people we had known and learned to love had been wonderfully supportive when Heather was alive and we really needed community support. I knew also, that the town officials and employees were also involved in the adoption process. They supported us with any requests we had made, often working late helping us to prepare documents so they would be ready early enough to get them to Boston for stamping. I could not imagine them being any different if and when we adopted a child.

After inspecting every inch of the house and the land around it, she finally gave a nod of approval, and we were on our way.

Chapter Thirty Two

In November of 1978, our caseworker called to invite us to a reception they were planning the following Sunday. It seemed Maria Cristina and her husband, Gustavo, were coming into Boston and they thought it would be nice if they got to meet with Maria Cristina's clients. Gustavo, I found out, was an architect, and had meetings with some of his American clients. Maria Cristina was tagging along, so to speak.

We picked up another couple from town who was also considering adoption and off we went to Boston. At the reception, I learned that out of the twenty or so couples there to meet Maria Cristina, we were perhaps nineteenth on the notorious list. I was crushed and went to the car to collect myself. Bruce, on the other hand, had gotten into a very animated conversation with Gustavo. By the time I got back in the room, they were the best of friends. It seemed they had flown into Boston earlier that morning and Maria Cristina was quite upset as all the stores were closed, and she really wanted to shop. This was, before the Blue Laws prohibiting Sunday openings had been repealed. Gustavo, who was fluent in English, was bemoaning the fact he only had a little time to take his wife shopping the next day, as he had to serve as her interpreter.

Bruce looked at him and said, "You know, we are in the women's clothing business, and we only live forty miles away. Why don't we see if Arlene can come into Boston tomorrow and take Maria Cristina and you straight to the distributors in town, and Maria Cristina can get whatever she likes at cost? Arlene will sign the invoices and when you're finished, you can add the totals of the invoices and send me a check."

After ten minutes of discussion and translating, it was decided I would pick them both up the following morning at nine am, and take Maria Cristina shopping.

As planned, I drove to the Hyatt in Cambridge the following morning, and picked them up. Gustavo had said he only had 90 minutes before his meeting, so we got straight to work.

Maria Cristina was like a kid at Disney-world. She had never seen so many clothes all in one building, and we went from floor to floor shopping. At 10:30, Gustavo called his appointment and postponed it to the following day. This was a once in a lifetime opportunity for them and they did not intend to waste a single minute of it. Maria Cristina proved to truly be a world class shopper. She devoted the entire day spending money and loving it. She'd try on a dress and parade around for Gustavo's and my benefit and approval. I had never seen a happier woman.

At 5:00 when I took them back to their hotel, all of us were exhausted. Gustavo added the total of all of the invoices and wrote a check for almost $10,000.

As we piled up all of the bundles and boxes for the doorman to take to their suite, Maria Cristina kissed me on both cheeks and said in broken English, "You will hear from us soon. We will see you again in Colombia, and it will be our pleasure to show you our beautiful city of Cali."

Chapter Thirty Three

December dragged. As we had mentioned to most of our friends we had decided to adopt, many of them did their best to try to be helpful. One friend called and said that she knew of an attorney in Ecuador who handled international adoptions and had contacted him on our behalf. He told her he had two sisters who had come up for adoption. One was six and the other was two. If we were interested, she said, she could contact the attorney and we could fly to Ecuador the next day and pick up the children.

I was ready to get on a plane the next morning. As determined as I was to go, that was how opposed Bruce was. He tried to talk some reason into me, but I was not interested. We were up all night battling about it. In the early morning hours, I finally came to my senses and understood how nonsensical this proposition truly was. None of the paperwork was done. There had to be more to it that simply flying down and taking two children home with me. Heartsick, I agreed to wait for Maria Cristina.

Chapter Thirty Four

January was cold and stormy, but not nearly as miserable as February. The span of two years time had not made February 10th any easier to live with. On that day, I went to the cemetery alone and wept by myself until I could no longer feel my hands or feet. Shivering, I went back to the car to warm up and compose myself enough to manage to drive home. That day was a black hole revisited. All of the memories flooded back, and I wallowed in a twenty-four hour long time warp. My dreams were palpable nightmares that had haunted me for two years following Heather's death. We all did the best we could and waited for the eleventh.

Alyssa was, by then, in the fourth grade and beginning to get some of her old confidence back. She too, had two long painful years to overcome. She was still taking her "piano lessons" and actually learning how to play the piano, but not well. She also continued with dance lessons and was becoming graceful and learning balance in all of her life. Of course, Cookie was her constant companion.

Late in February, I got a call from Gustavo, who was translating for Maria Cristina.

"Congratulations," he said, "You have a son." I was shocked. To the best of our knowledge, none of the other families in the Colombian program had been placed with children. We had magically jumped to the top of the list.

"We did not call you sooner," he continued, "because the baby was premature and Maria Cristina wanted to be sure that the baby was all right. But, you have a beautiful son, and he looks just like your family." I did not understand his remark about the baby looking just like us, but I was too stunned to question it.

"Your son was born February 11." When he said that, I nearly fell on the floor. It was two years and one day after Heather died.

" He is two and a half months premature and is very small, but very healthy, and now you can begin to do the things you need to do before you come to Colombia. With luck, we will see you some time in April. Congratulations again, on the birth of your son."

We no sooner hung up the phone than it rang again. This time it was International Adoptions. They were flabbergasted and furious. When Maria Cristina had notified them, she said this baby was specifically for us and was not to go to anyone else. She had been adamant in her decision and there was nothing that they could say to convince her the baby should go to one of the other families who had been waiting longer than we had. She would discuss it no more. Either we got this baby, or else. They were enraged. The baby had all ready been given the name Gregory Hayden, the reversed form of the name we had chosen for a boy, on his birth certificate, and there was nothing to be done to change it. When we heard this, we too were amazed, but we did understand it.

We were elated by the news. Alyssa ran around the house screaming and yelling, "I have a baby brother!!! I have a baby brother!!!" I remember calling Carl and Sylvia and they were also thrilled, finally, after five granddaughters, a boy in the family. Then I called my mother. She too was thrilled. Her reactions, however, were a little unusual.

When she asked me "Are both of his parents Jewish?"

I answered, "Yes, we both are."

When she asked, "College graduates?"

Again I answered, "yes we both are."

But when she asked "Is this child going to be able to speak English?" I lost it, and reverted to smart-mouth again, and told her, "No, I thought that we'd raise him to speak fluent Chinese." That ended that conversation.

The following weeks were a blur. We had to apply for an entrance visa for the baby. This meant back and forth to Boston to get the paperwork prepared. We had to gather all of the necessary documents, papers and parcels. In one of her letters, Maria Cristina told us things would be a lot easier and transpire more smoothly, if we brought small gifts appropriate for either a man or a woman, to be used as "tokens of gratitude" for making the process as easy as possible in Colombia. In other words, our tokens of gratitude were small tokens of bribery for not making things any more complicated than they needed to be. These were to be used for the clerks in the courts, the secretaries and the judges as well, in the Colombian system. We had to finalize the adoption in Cali, before we could take the baby out of the country.

Also, we had to prepare for traveling with an infant, and to prepare our home. We had given away all of our baby things after Heather had been born, as we had expected no further children. All of those items had to be purchased again. We had to get a crib, stroller, changing table, dresser and all of the other accoutrements needed by infants and get them in place in what was to have been Heather's room. We picked out wallpaper, all bright red, blue and green football players and team names. There was so much to do and so little time.

Alyssa opted not to fly to Colombia with us. I think that she probably would have come if the US Public Health Service had not recommended shots for Typhoid, Yellow Fever, Tetanus and a revaccination for Small Pox. When she saw the laundry list of inoculations, she decided to stay at home.

Since we were planning to travel during the school calendar, we decided to accept the gracious invitation of our next door neighbors, Sue and Mike Wildfeuer, for Lyssa to stay at their house. Had Alyssa chosen to stay with her grandparents in Worcester, they would have had to drive her back and forth to school every day. Also, she wanted to be able to go home every morning and afternoon to look after Cookie.

Our travel date April 19 was rapidly approaching and we were no where near ready. The visa had not been prepared as of April 10th and we were beginning to panic. Slowly and carefully we compiled our documents, gifts and baby things to travel. We had purchased a large straw baby basket to use as a travel bed for the baby. It was lined with red calico and had a canopy on the top to keep the sun off the baby's head. This we stuffed with Pampers, bottles, clothes and an immersion coil to use whenever we had to boil water.

John Tkach had suggested we keep him on whatever diet they had used in the nursery in Cali. He thought that we would have enough trouble without having to change diets in a foreign country. On top of all of this, International Adoptions asked us to take a few things down for the orphanage they used whenever their babies were not in private nurseries, as was ours. Their few things were, in reality, fifteen cartons of food, clothes, appliances, medical supplies and diapers. These, they had packed and had waiting at Worcester Airport for us to take to Colombia.

We had to fly from Worcester, to La Guardia, then take a very large cab to Kennedy for our Avianca flight to Bogota. When we arrived at Kennedy, schlepping all of our baggage, plus the cartons International Adoptions had sent along, the attendant at the Avianca desk went nuts. They had agreed to transport a few boxes, not all of this. They called Boston, and screamed at the administrator of the agency for about twenty minutes, then swearing in Spanish, agreed to take the bundles, one last time. International Adoptions was told never to do that again. We promised, with full assurance, we would never have any part in doing something like this again. Now at least, the cartons were taken off of our hands.

We finally boarded our flight on Avianca'a one and only Jumbo Jet and took off for Bogota.

Chapter Thirty Five

No sooner had the plane taken off, than the flight crew switched from English to Spanish. All of the flight information they gave us was in Spanish, and all that we could do was try not to listen, and focus on the baby.

When we landed in Bogota, it was more like landing in a demilitarized zone, than into friendly territory. The airport was heavily patrolled by Colombian Militiamen all armed with bayoneted rifles.

We had three hours to kill until our flight to Cali. During that time we had to clear Colombian customs. We claimed our luggage and the proceeded to an area that looked as though it had been bombed during the London Blitz. There were large, menacing German Shepherds roaming around with their handlers, sniffing all of the baggage for contraband drugs. We no longer had to worry about the parcels from International Adoptions, as International Adoptions had arranged for their handling, but the customs agents went through every single item we had. They opened and thumbed through each Pamper, bottle and item of baby clothing. I remember wondering if they were this careful when one left the country.

After the customs agents and dogs finished with our luggage, we were approached by a porter who spoke broken English, and offered to carry all of our bags from the International terminal to the National terminal where we could get our flight from Bogota to Cali five American dollars. We counter offered three and he agreed. He then picked up our luggage and carried it the twenty feet, from International to National. That was our first lesson about life in Colombia.

Next, we went to a small cafe in the airport to get some cold drinks. We ordered two Coca Colas and eventually were served, after we finally succeeded in making ourselves understood. Not an easy task. Bruce gave the waitress a one-dollar bill. We received no change, and assumed the Cokes were fifty cents each and would leave a tip when we left.

As we were sitting there looking very bewildered another American asked if he could join us. As we had met him on the plane, we said, "Sure". He also ordered a Coke, but in Spanish. He gave the waitress a dime, and got back a nickel in change. Slowly, we were beginning to get it. This was how it was done in Colombia.

Fortunately, he told us what gate we needed to find for our commuter flight to Cali. Since he had a later flight, he graciously escorted us to the waiting area. He wished us luck (obviously we looked like we needed all of the luck we could get), and went to his flight.

The flight between Bogota and Cali, is a short commuter hop straight up over the Andes, and then almost straight down again. It was customary for commuters in Colombia to try to get onto earlier flights if they had finished with their business before their scheduled flights. When we boarded, we had to have the flight attendant kick two people out of our seats and tell them to leave the plane. Many of these commuters refused to leave, and chose instead to stand in the aisles. One man, who adamantly refused to leave the plane, rode in the cockpit. Although I had never been a nervous flyer before, since that flight, I have joined the ranks of the white-knuckle fliers society.

The plane finally got off the ground, 45 minutes late (as was everything in Colombia), and we flew to Cali. The man sitting across the aisle from us was also American. He said this flight crowding was common practice in Colombia. He worked for an American pharmaceutical company in Cali, and lightly quipped that this flight almost always eventually made the trip without consequence. I was not sure if he was kidding or not.

Chapter Thirty Six

When we landed a half-hour later and took a taxi to the hotel we were staying at. As confused as I had thought the airline and airport was the traffic and road system made it look like a model of speed and efficiency. There had been an accident in an intersection and four directions of traffic were halted. Cars were driving on embankments trying to avoid the hold up. At one point our cab was almost hanging off the easement of the road as our cabby tried to navigate into Cali. Traffic stopped for cows that strolled in the pastures that flanked the roads. I had never seen anything like it.

Maria Cristina and Gustavo met us at the door of the hotel. We hugged and kissed, like long lost friends. By this time, we had been traveling for more than seventeen hours and we were exhausted. Maria Cristina had booked us into the finest hotel in Cali, and it was quite beautiful. It also was surrounded by a twelve-foot high brick wall, and conspicuously well guarded by rifled militiamen. Our room was not ready, and Maria Cristina yelled and carried on at the desk clerk about his lack of professionalism, and then told us that she and Gustavo wanted us to be their guests for dinner, outside poolside in the hotel's patio restaurant. What else could we say, but yes.

It was at dinner, Maria Cristina, through Gustavo, told us everything that we needed to know and explained to us about the political unrest in Colombia. This was, she explained, with Gustavo's help, a society of two classes, filthy rich and dirt poor. Things were very volatile and there had been threats. Also, the wife of the President of Colombia was staying at this hotel. Hence, the extra security. She told us we had nothing to worry about as long as we did not go out of the hotel alone after dark. I remember thinking to myself, "not a chance in Hell that is going to happen."

When we finished eating, our room was ready and they kissed us both good-bye and said to be ready at 8:00am sharp, the following morning to see the baby. Although we were both exhausted, neither one of us slept much that night. We were up for breakfast at 6:00am and waited in the lobby at 8:00. Gustavo was there to pick us up promptly at 8:45. We drove across town to pick up Maria Cristina and then to see the baby.

When we got to the nursery where he had been since being discharged from the clinica where he had been born, we found it to be beautiful and immaculate. A smiling, round-faced, large black woman went upstairs and came down with our child. He was dressed in a white hand crocheted saque that had been embroidered with blue and green flowers. There were also hand crocheted booties and a hat. He was so small it was hard to imagine that he was almost three months old. The single most amazing thing happened when we looked at his face. He looked almost identical to both Alyssa and Heather when they had been infants. He looked just like Bruce.

This wasn't just a vague resemblance he really looked like one of our natural children. It was scary, how closely he resembled Heather in particular. We were both in a state of shock.

For some reason I was under the impression that we would see the baby, then do some paper work and go back and pick him up afterwards, but I was wrong. After seeing the baby for the first time and being so startled, I felt like I needed some time to decompress. But there was no time, he was ours from that first second that we picked him up and held him.

When at last, we composed ourselves and everyone had finished with congratulations and thank-yous all around, we signed the necessary paperwork and were told we were free to go. When I asked about what foods they were feeding him they told me the name of the infant formula, and then said he was also being fed orange juice and strained pears. Having fed two other infants, I was shocked again at their choice of diet for this tiny, eight pound, three-month-old baby. I smiled, however, and thanked them again for taking such wonderful and loving care of my child. By that time, I was learning how to play the game in Colombia, and said nothing about what I considered to be a totally inappropriate choice of diet for an infant.

Chapter Thirty Seven

Gustavo then drove us to a market so I could purchase some baby food and formula. He had to come into the store with me so I could locate and pay for the items I needed. I came out with three large containers of dry infant formula, a tin of banana flakes and two boxes of rice cereal. No more orange juice and pears for this child. Then Gustavo drove us back to the hotel, and wished us well. He said he would pick us up, with the baby, that night so we could all have dinner together. He assured us the baby nurse they had for their children would be happy to look after our baby for us while we had dinner. Then he left us alone to really meet and get to know

our new son, who we had all ready started to call Greg.

This was an amazing experience. When we got settled in and looked him over from head to toe we realized just how much this child looked like one of our own.

At one point I turned to Bruce and asked," So, what were you doing in Colombia a year ago?"

He was as shocked as I was at the resemblance. Greg was a very tiny, but alert and happy baby. He was comfortable with us immediately and smiled all of the time. As were both Alyssa and Heather, Greg was dark haired with enormous black eyes. He was complexioned as was Alyssa with a medium olive tone skin, and had dimples in all of the same places that Heather had. His facial structure was almost identical to Alyssa's, and his mouth and nose were shaped as Heather's had been. It was an eerie resemblance to Heather in particular, and we were both a little dazed and startled by the similarities.

Greg was, however a much better natured baby than were either of the girls at the same age. When we went out of the room, we would pack him into the baby basket and tuck him in with a silky blanket and pacifier, and he would comfortably travel with us wherever we went.

When we had to go to court, invariably he would charm all of the office staff, and they happily offered to play and watch him as we sat in a judge's chambers listening and smiling and not understanding a single word of what was happening around us. When the court session was over, we graciously thanked the judge and the clerks and gave them each a small gift that we had brought with us for these exact situations. They would say "Gracias" and all of our paperwork was then processed swiftly and without a hitch.

When we were not in court or doing paperwork, we were free to walk around the city, sightseeing and shopping. We found that for $2. American money, an English speaking cab driver would take us where ever we wanted to go, then wait for us and drive us back and forth to the hotel for an entire day. During one of our shopping excursions, we met a woman who owned a shop in one of the more exclusive sections of the city. As she spoke fluent English, we struck an immediate friendship. She told us she owned the shop and ran the business, while her husband managed their family owned sugar plantation. She also mentioned that she did charity work helping unwed mothers through a church group, and she was very well connected. She offered to find out, for us, if we wished, any information that might be available about the baby. We thanked her, and told her all we wanted to know was if the birth parents were normal and healthy, and if there were any special medical problems we should know about.

She said she would try to find out some information for us, and asked us to meet her the following afternoon at her shop.

When we returned the next afternoon, after pouring coffee for us, she told us what she had been able to learn. All she could find out was that his birth mother had been fifteen when she delivered. She was healthy and had no obvious medical problems. The girl's pregnancy had been an embarrassment for her upper class parents. It was they who had surrendered the baby for adoption. Both Bruce and I were relieved to hear this good news, and to show our appreciation; we invited her to join us for dinner that night at the rooftop restaurant at our hotel. She agreed.

When we met at nine that evening, at the elevator leading up to the roof, Greg was happily sleeping in his basket. His basket rested on a chair between Bruce and me as we ate. She sat across from us. As we had dinner we talked about our families, and before we knew it, she looked at her watch and announced, "It is eleven o'clock. My bodyguard is waiting for me downstairs." Shocked by this revelation, we asked her to call downstairs to say she would be a little late.

When she returned to our table, she further explained that she was from a very wealthy family. Both her grandmother and her uncle had been kidnapped and held for ransom. She never traveled anywhere without an armed escort. We were stunned. We had never realized how bad the situation was, or how desperate were the people of Colombia. Before she left for the evening, she asked us to stop at her store one more time before we left Cali.

In the morning of the day that we were flying from Cali to Bogota, we stopped at her shop. She gave me a small-carved stone replica of a god from one of the Indian ruins in Colombia. It was, she said, a piece from her family's collection and she hoped that it would serve as a pleasant reminder of our stay in Cali. She further advised us to pack the stone statue carefully, when leaving the country, as the Colombian customs agents did not look favorably on tourists leaving with antiquities. We kissed each other good bye and said our thanks to her.

We had spent eight days in Cali with Maria Cristina and Gustavo as our gracious hosts, and then flew back to Bogota to finish up all of the paperwork that had to be handled through the American Embassy.

Bogota in April reminded me of Manhattan in February. The skies were steel gray, and the streets not terribly inviting. The temperature hovered about the 45degree mark, a distinct difference from the balmy 80s of Cali. On the ninth day, in Bogota, we were all sick with vomiting and diarrhea. Greg screamed with stomach cramps, and Bruce and I were not fit to do much of anything. We had to go to the American Embassy and have the final paperwork completed. The Embassy building looked like an armed fortress. There were Marines with side arms at the gates, and at each doorway. Finally, we were permitted through the heavy vault like doors, to the inside of the Embassy. Never, had either of us conceived of the security measures that had to be taken to keep the Embassy secure. Literally, at the last possible minute, less than an hour before the Embassy closed, we completed the paperwork. We were now free to take an alien into the United States.

Returning to the hotel, Bruce and I felt marginally better, and decided that we were never coming back to Bogota, and if we wanted to look around, this was the time. We packed Greg in his basket, and set out on foot to explore the radius of the Intercontinental Hotel in Bogota.

Packs of children and teenagers roved the streets begging for money. We learned early, that when we gave change to these children, a new pack would pick up the scent and follow us begging for more. We went into an underground shopping mall, beneath the hotel, and wandered around there for a short while, before seeing a bearded man, sitting at one end of the mall, with a shotgun in his lap. It was his job, we found out, to shoot thieves.

By the morning of the tenth day, we were all sick and miserable and just wanted to be out of Colombia. It did not matter how badly we felt, we drank Pepto Bismol and got a cab to Bogota airport.

When we got there, we had to be searched by the

Colombian Police. The men went into one room and the women and children into another, where we were frisked and sniffed by dogs and our luggage was inspected carefully. They went through all of Greg's baby things and searched the bottom and lining of the baby basket. Luckily they did not look into Greg's diaper, and did not notice the small plastic bag carrying our souvenir. Our flight was then delayed, because Avianca Airlines was filming a television commercial using their one and only 747 Jumbo Jet, the one we were ready to board.

Once airborne, we were so exhausted we slept until they announced the arrival at Miami International Airport.

After deplaning we had to go through American customs and get cleared through the agriculture department, where the USDA representative confiscated all of Greg's formula. There had been a reported outbreak of Hoof and Mouth Disease among Colombian dairy cattle. No dairy products were allowed into the United States. As much as I complained about taking the baby's food away, they did not want to hear about it, and they took all the tins of dry milk anyway.

By that time, we were in the International Arrivals area of Miami International terminal with a screaming, hungry baby, who had no formula to drink. Schlepping all of our luggage, souvenirs and a hysterical infant in a wicker basket, we had to try to locate a pharmacy where we could purchase some pre-bottled Similac and a package of nipples. Then we had to try to get to the National Departures area in time to make our flight back to Boston.

Bruce and I were both ready to collapse. Neither of us knew how far the National terminal was from where we were, but it seemed like miles. When we finally got there, I remember sitting in the lounge outside the Delta departure area, half dead and running into a friend from home who was also waiting for our flight. I watched in amazement as Bruce and our friend actually ate hot dogs and drank pina coladas and thought Bruce should have his head examined for eating that combination. But he swears, to this day, it was the hot dog and pina colada that cured his

Montezuma's Revenge. I can't say that even the smell of it, did me any good.

Except for Greg's screaming non-stop from Miami to Boston, our flight was uneventful. Carl and Sylvia met us at Logan Airport in Boston. When we finally arrived at home at 11:30 on the night of April 30th 1979, Alyssa came back home with Mike and Sue Wildfeuer to meet her new baby brother for the first time. As the Wildfeuers came into the house to greet us, Mike had a copy of Time Magazine, folded in the middle. He showed us a picture of the police station in Cali. It had been bombed by terrorists while we were in Cali. Not understanding Spanish, we had no idea anything like that had happened while we were there. It was good to be home.

Chapter Thirty Eight

Alyssa immediately took over with Greg, as she was now an expert on infant care, learning everything she needed to know from watching the girls with the Luftig's baby son, Micah. It was love at first sight between the two of them. She called all of her girlfriends over the next day to show off her new baby. Five days later, we had the Bris. Greg met the rest of his family and new friends that day. More than one hundred people crowded into our house to celebrate. Greg was ritually circumcised and prayed over and had taken the first step before being converted to Judaism. Although he did not have a particularly good time that day, the rest of us had a ball. Carl's friend Jack Pearl catered the entire event. Sharon Luftig was his god-mother. There was ease and naturalness in the way that Greg fit into the family. He was home.

Chapter Thirty Nine

We have been family: normal, relatively healthy most of the time, and very happy since. The childhood problems and illnesses that Greg had were never more serious than a series of ear infections that led to tubes being inserted. The real crisis days had passed. It was never our intention to replace one child with another, clearly that is an impossible task. What we did, was rebuild on the ruins of a totally devastated family. But, in short, it was our only method of survival. Sometimes there is life after death.

Aftermath

Since we've been together this long, I think you need to be brought up to date on how we are doing.

Greg became a naturalized citizen in April 1980. His American adoption was finalized shortly thereafter. He was a happy and healthy child. He had the usual childhood problems, and surgery twice two put tubes in his ears to correct a slight hearing problem. Always being very small for his age, he also was diagnosed with a growth disorder when he was seven. At eight years of age, he started taking growth hormone injections, and now at the tender and frequently obnoxious age of twenty one, he is five feet eight inches tall, strong, handsome, happy and driving us all nuts. In other words, he is a perfectly normal kid.

Alyssa blossomed and grew. She was Student Council President in her Junior High School class. She danced with beauty, vigor and passion until she injured her knees at age sixteen, and had to have surgery. She went to Syracuse University and then received her Jurist Doctor degree from the New England School of Law in May of 1994. She too, is healthy and happy. She is the director of Career Services at the New England School of Law in Boston. April 19, 1997 she married Eric Hammond. They are expecting their first child, a little girl, in January 2001.

My mother in law, Sylvia died in 1982. Carl died in 1993. They are both deeply missed. Carl enjoyed a beautiful relationship with all of his grandchildren, but there was always a special fondness and attachment for his one and only grandson, Greg.

My mother is well, happy and now living in assisted living in Massachusetts. She too, is close to all of her grandchildren, but dotes especially on her youngest grandchild, Greg.

The Luftigs moved to South Carolina in 1983, then to Louisiana. I miss them all, very much.

Sue and Mike Wildfeuer lived next door until 1997 when they retired to Florida. I could not have had better next door neighbors.

Bruce, Greg and I still live in Paxton, sharing our home with one cat and two Yorkshire Terrorists, sorry I mean Terriers.

The woman's clothing business is still there, as is Bruce. He is older, wiser, grayer, thicker in the middle and a little more tired than he used to be, but basically the same guy.

I am the same, but a little older and a little wiser. Forever changed by circumstance and luck, I am a whole lot smarter, and a whole lot dumber.

As for the rest of it, about six months after we adopted Greg, I met Jean Whitcomb at the town pharmacy.

She smiled and said," Tell Alyssa to stick to dancing, she really isn't very good at the piano."

THE END